LETHAL LOZENGES AND TAINTED TEA:

A BIOGRAPHY OF JOHN POSTGATE (1820-1881)

by
John Postgate

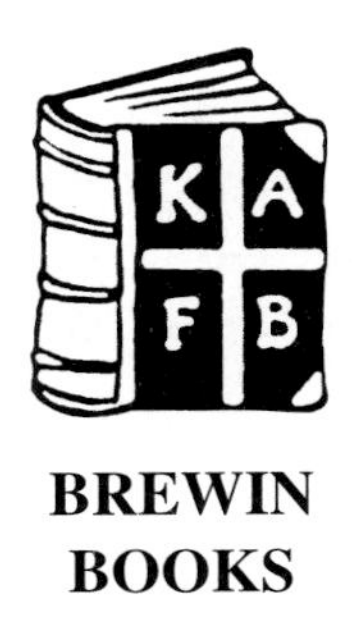

BREWIN
BOOKS

First published in 2001 by
Brewin Books, Studley, Warwickshire B80 7LG

British Library Cataloguing in Publication Data
A catalogue record for this book is available from
The British Library

ISBN: 1 85858 178 8

Typeset in Plantin and made and printed
in Great Britain by Warwick Printing Company Limited,
Theatre Street, Warwick, Warwickshire CV34 4DR.

CONTENTS

ILLUSTRATIONS

PREFACE

Professor John Postgate FRCS (1820-81), the present writer's great-grandfather, was a Victorian reformer who dedicated the greater part of his adult life to a crusade against the practice, widespread in his day, of adulterating food and drugs. The story of his ultimate success, the passage through Parliament of the Food and Drug Adulteration Acts of the mid nineteenth century, was a remarkable cliff-hanger of which I only became aware when writing the biography of his grandson [0.1]. At the same time I discovered the considerable extent to which that contribution to social reform in Victorian Britain, and hence to our well-being today, had been forgotten.

It had not been entirely forgotten, however. In a study of drug adulteration in Victorian Britain published in 1966 [0.2] E W Steib wrote of John Postgate, "A definitive biography of this important figure is needed". In this attempt to meet that need I have collated what I could discover of his personality and background, and tried to clarify his part in the history of this strange patch of turbulence in the flow of mid-Victorian reforms. Definitive material has been far from abundant, because the papers he bequeathed to a descendant have disappeared [0.3]. My most fruitful sources have been Dr James Langford's (1887) chronicle of mid nineteenth-century Birmingham [0.4]; an anonymous biographical sketch of John Postgate in *The Biograph & Review* for 1880 [0.5]; and an admirable but little-known attempt to restore Postgate's credentials published by the Birmingham historian B T Davis in 1967 [0.6].

The *dramatis personae* include several exceptional and idiosyncratic personalities, but my accounts of them in the main text have been restricted in order to keep my narrative focussed on Postgate himself. I have provided more detailed information, with appropriate references, in the 'notes and references' section.

....

I am grateful to Dr Margaret Gelling OBE FBA for helpful advice and an invaluable tour of Birmingham, and to my wife Mary for carefully reading and checking the text of this book. I also thank the Royal Society for a grant to assist its publication.

Emeritus Professor John Postgate FRS — Lewes, 2000

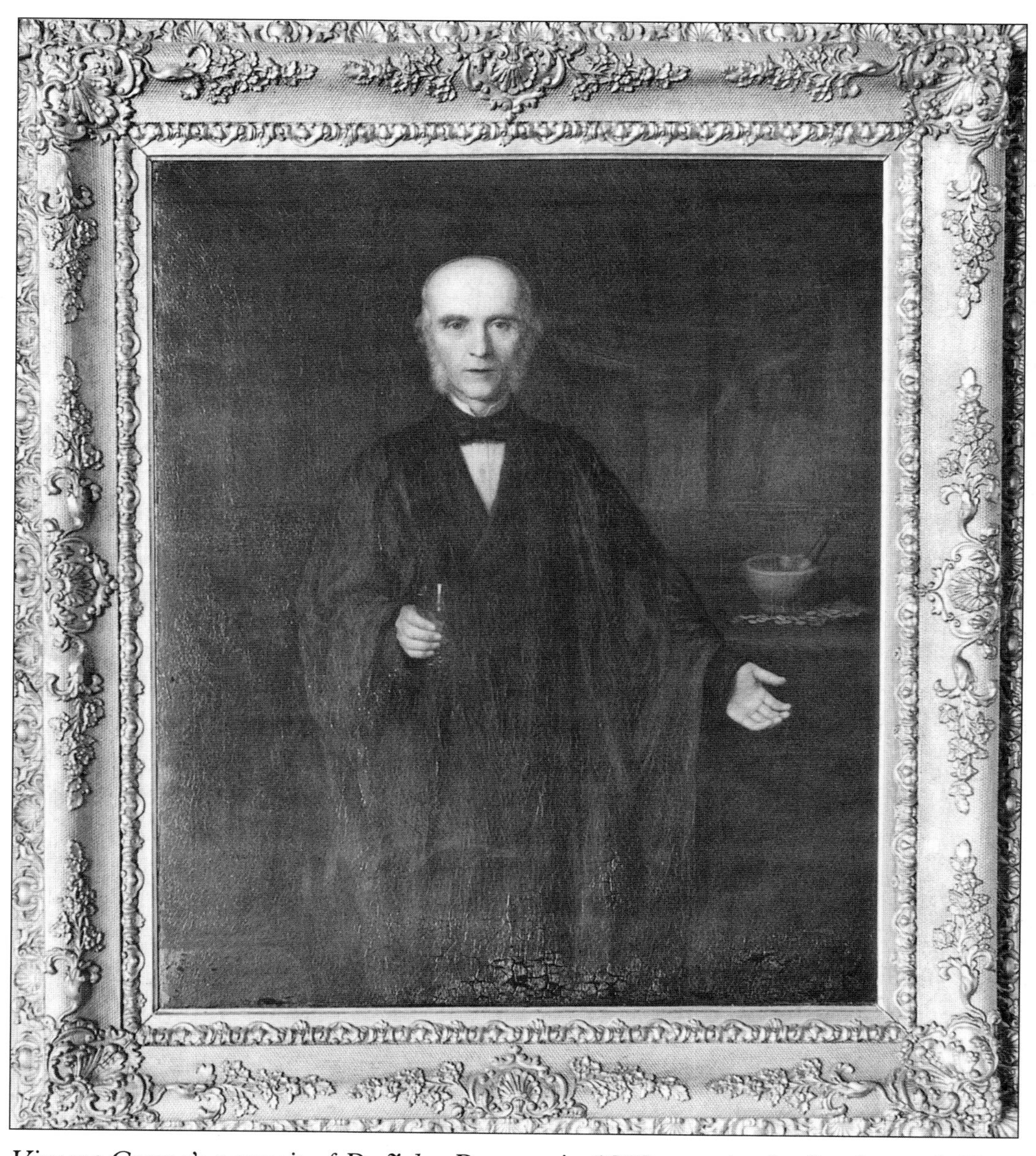

Vincent Crome's portrait of Dr John Postgate in 1878, now in the Scarborough Town Hall (courtesy of the Scarborough Borough Council).

Chapter 1

THE BACKGROUND

The adulteration of merchandise must be quite as old as commerce itself. It amounts to fooling or defrauding the customer for profit, by manipulating a commodity so that it appears to be purer, or of better quality, than it really is. The coal merchant who takes care to bag-up his smokeless fuel after rain, when it is heavy with damp; the greengrocer who scoops a little soil into a bag of 'organic' potatoes; the North African sandal vendor whose lovely hand-worked leather proves to conceal layered cardboard: these are present-day examples of a tradition of commercial deception that goes back into remote history. Irritating to the deluded customer, no doubt, but these are mild examples, on that indistinct borderline which separates deliberate carelessness from intentional dishonesty. However, traders' frauds have not always been so gentle; some, such as the debasing of precious metals or the faking of precious stones, can amount to theft on a grand scale; others, such as the down-grading of building materials or the adulteration of food, drink and medicine, can be dangerous and even life-threatening.

Sharing food is an integral and essential element of our social lives – this truism applies to all societies, from the most primitive to the most complex. We take for granted the consequence that the number of people involved in victualling – by which I mean those who grow, hunt, gather, distribute, prepare or serve food – is always smaller than the number of people who consume it. As societies have evolved from hunter-gatherers towards the complex and technology-based societies of today, progressively fewer and fewer of the total population of consumers work in the victualling network. Today, from farmyard to kitchen, elaborate and highly automated systems have been developed for the primary production of food and drink, for their storage, distribution and processing, even for their serving. This social diversification is in many ways a splendid thing, and it has greatly enhanced the quality of modern life, but inevitably it has opened up numerous opportunities for fraud, deception and malfeasance. We are, some say regrettably, nothing if not human, and there have always been those who will seize such opportunities, perhaps for personal gain, perhaps out of laziness, occasionally because of malevolence or simple stupidity.

Civilised communities have recognised the possibility of fraud by adulteration for many centuries, and have generally expected their governments to protect the customer [1.1, 1.2]. Understandably, it is the adulteration of food, drink and medicines that has been the foremost source of public anxiety.

Herodotus recorded that in pre-Hellenic Thasos (in the 6th century BC) the highly esteemed wine of this Aegean island had to be brought to the agora for sale in sealed vessels. It was a strong, heavy wine to which customers would normally add water before drinking, but heavy fines were levied on merchants found guilty of selling it already watered. Again, ancient Athens and Rome employed official inspectors whose duties were to monitor laws against the flavouring and colouring of wine. In the medical context, Pedacius Dioscoredes, a Greek surgeon of the first century AD, compiled a *De Materia Medica* which included, among over 1000 entries, forty instances of adulterated materials plus, for many, descriptions of ways of detection. The Roman physician Galen (129-201 AD) also criticised drug dealers for supplying adulterated products.

In England, records of regulation go back to the reign of Edward The Confessor (1042-66), when a knavish brewer of Chester was punished by being dragged through the streets in a cart containing what an Edwardian writer politely termed "the residues of the local privies". In 1203, King John (1199-1216) proclaimed regulations regarding bakers' bread, and in 1266, under his successor Henry III (1216-72), a statute concerning food quality was promulgated, threatening dishonest bakers, brewers, vintners, butchers and others with "the pillory and tumbril". As cited during the reign of Edward I (1272-1307), the statute concerning bread prescribed shaming punishments for transgressors:

> "If any default be found in the bread of a baker in the city, the first time, let him be drawn on a hurdle from the Guildhall to his own house through the great street where there be most people assembled, and through the great streets which are most dirty, with the faulty loaf hanging from his neck; if a second time he shall be found committing the same offence, let him be drawn from the Guildhall through the great street of Cheepe in the manner aforesaid to the pillory, and let him be put upon the pillory, and let him remain there at least one hour in the day; and the third time that such a default be found, he shall be drawn, and the oven shall be pulled down, and the baker made to foreswear the trade in the city for ever."

During the reign of Charles I (1625-49), in 1634, the statute was widened to include the sale of "musty or corrupt" foodstuffs, prescribing comparable imaginative punishments, and it remained in force until its repeal in 1709 under Queen Anne (1702-14).

In addition to the law-enforcement authorities, the mediaeval Guilds and later the City Companies had a duty to maintain the quality and purity of the goods their members dealt in, and additional legislation had been introduced at intervals after 1266 to help them discharge this duty. For example, in the seventeenth century the Apothecaries' Company had the power to inspect apothecaries' shops, and if adulterated goods were found the stock would be burned in the street outside the shop and the vendor punished, perhaps by being expelled from the Company. (Steib [1.3] recorded that punishments could be even more severe in Europe: "in mediaeval Nürnberg, several adulterers of saffron had been burned along with their adulterated goods".) But it seems to be true of Britain that, although a few miscreants were summoned and punished, the legislation was largely ineffective. There was a good reason, of course: policing such fraud was not at all easy until the era of proper chemical and biological analyses. The major tests then available made use of taste, smell, texture and general appearance – properties that could often be faked quite easily. Not that the fraudsters had everything their own way. According to City records, 'ale tasters', employed under Edward the Confessor to check on brewers, would test ale by spilling some on a wooden seat, sitting on the wet place in their leather breeches and judging the stickiness of the drying residue; if the ale had been sugared, the taster would stick to the seat. Around 1550, 'five pipes' of wine were ordered to be destroyed by the Lord Mayor of London because of a kind of retrospective analysis: bundles of weeds, pieces of sulphur match and "a kind of gravel mixture sticking to the casks" were found when the wine was racked off.

Tea was introduced into Britain around 1660 and as its popularity spread down the social classes during the eighteenth century, it seems to have become curiously susceptible to adulteration. It was the subject of a succession of enactments; one in 1730-31 proscribed its adulteration with dyes, liquorice leaves, sloe leaves, used-and-dried tea leaves, the leaves of other shrubs and trees, sugar, molasses, clay or logwood; the penalties included fines and imprisonment.

The existence of published *materia medica* and, in the nineteenth century, of pharmacopoeias, together with some control exerted by the Apothecaries' Company and, after 1841, the Pharmaceutical Society, seem to have contained the adulteration of drugs to a limited extent. However, despite legislation, and despite occasional protests, pamphlets or broadsheets (mainly emanating from physicians), food and drink adulteration remained a common hazard of everyday life throughout the eighteenth and well into the nineteenth centuries. Mrs Beeton, in the first edition of her famous *Book of Household Management* (1861) [1.4] warned almost casually that "sugar is adulterated with fine sand and sawdust" and more firmly that, "This rage for white bread has introduced adulterations of a very serious character...", mentioning potato flour as a "comparatively harmless cheat" and alum and bone dust as "far from harmless" additives. In the late eighteenth century the more honest grocers employed 'garblers', whose duty was to remove gross foreign matter such as stones and dust from spices which were to be sold.

Bread seems to have been another especially vulnerable commodity. As well as the potato flour, alum and bone dust of Mrs Beeton's warning, its recorded adulterants included bean meal, bone ash or meal, chalk, sand and slaked lime. Alum was added as a bleaching agent; a crooked baker might expect to get away with adding sand or ash because grit from the millstone was a natural hazard in flour. Coffee, like tea, came into use in the seventeenth century, and was also especially susceptible to adulteration. Among proscribed additives were grass, burned or scorched acorns, roasted chicory and, curiously, butter or lard. Gravel, leaves and twigs might be added to pepper and, after about 1650, clove dust too. Mustard would be diluted with wheatflour, pea flour, radish seeds or cayenne pepper. Sugar, which came into prominence as a foodstuff in the 1500s, was not only likely to contain sand or sawdust, but was usually poorly refined. Lead salts would be used to clarify wine, though their toxicity had been recognized for several centuries. And, of course, the customer had always to be alert in case beer, milk or wine should prove to have been diluted with water, an adulterant which, albeit unwelcome, was at least not toxic.

Although the majority of additives were quite simply fraudulent and often dangerous, it is interesting that a few in due course became established components of prepared foods. Thus the use of hops to add bitterness to beer was regarded as fraudulent in the fifteenth century, but is now universal practice; and all over Europe, especially in France, people enjoy, even prefer, coffee which contains that erstwhile adulterant, chicory. In New Orleans, USA, such coffee has become an admired speciality of the French Quarter.

To-day Western societies take for granted government responsibility for the quality of food, and expect government to discharge that responsibility with the utmost seriousness. But it was not always so; it required some strong-minded Georgians and Victorians to ensure that Parliament not only accepted its responsibility towards the consumer but acted upon it. One of those campaigners was John Postgate FRCS of Birmingham [1.5;1.6].

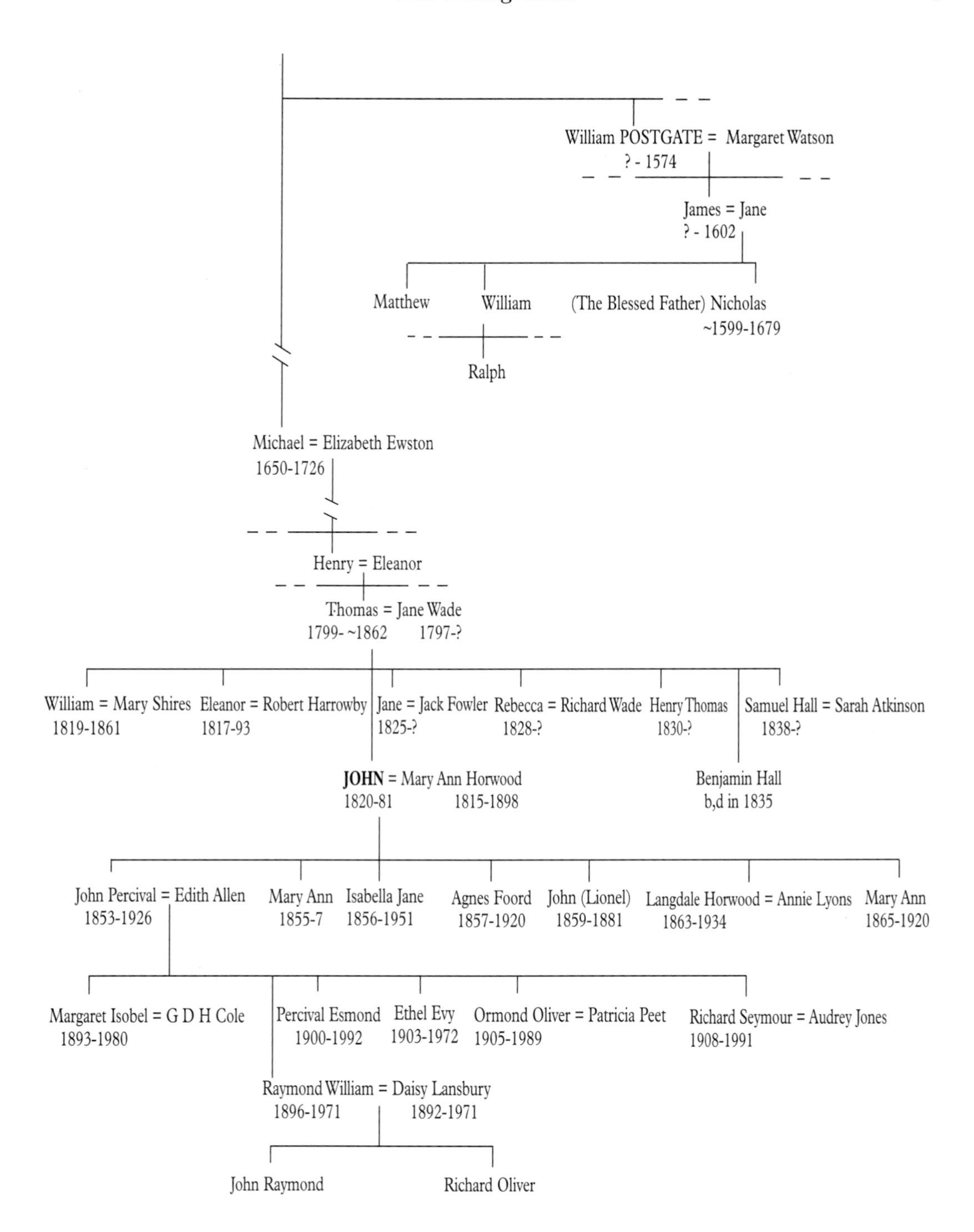

ABRIDGED FAMILY TREE

(Broken lines of descent indicate uncertain genealogy; dashed lines mean siblings, if any, not traced)

Chapter 2

EARLY DAYS

The Postgates were of Yorkshire stock [2.1]. John Postgate was born at Scarborough, on the Yorkshire coast, on 21 October 1820. He was a son of Thomas Postgate, a joiner and sometime builder and auctioneer. Thomas's father was Henry Postgate, also a Scarborough builder, whose wife was Eleanor (maiden name unknown). Family tradition has it that a collateral ancestor was Father Nicholas Postgate of Egton Bridge, a local priest still widely remembered by Yorkshire Catholics. Father Nicholas was beatified in the 1980s, having had the unfortunate distinction of being among the very last British Roman Catholic martyrs [2.2]. John's genealogy (see the accompanying tree, amplified in notes 2.2 and 2.3) is insecure as far as Father Nicholas is concerned, but from Henry onwards it has documentary support.

According to parish records and the periodic census, several families of Postgates, presumably more or less related to each other, lived along the North Yorkshire coast and in the Eskdale villages, and the menfolk from Whitby and Scarborough were often seafarers. Thomas and his family resided at No. 9, Old Cliffe Road, Scarborough (the street no longer exists), and he seems to have sired a clan of distinctive personalities [2.3]. Parish records together with the will of John's father indicate that Thomas's wife Jane, *née* Wade, presented him with nine offspring in all. John was their third child; eight survived into adulthood, but Benjamin Hall, their penultimate child, died in his first year; a cousin, Louise Wade, was raised as part of the family.

Scarborough at the beginning of the nineteenth century was a prosperous town. Its main industry was shipbuilding; there were 11 yards engaged principally in building the coastal colliers which transported coal from the Northern pits to the South of Britain. Shipbuilding supported much ancillary employment such as work with iron and timber suppliers, with manufacturers of rope walks and ladders, sail lofts etc. A small fishing industry was growing, but Scarborough's best-known source of wealth was as a health resort, servicing visitors and holidaymakers drawn to the town by the reputation of its spa water.

In 1626 a Mistress Farrow had discovered a spring producing restorative water located below the South Cliff, and visitors soon came from far and near to drink its water, drawn from a public well. In 1698 part of the cliff collapsed dramatically, and the resulting landslide, taking with it a herd of cattle, obliterated the spring. Though it was soon rediscovered, it then remained inaccessible for over a century. However, Scarborough remained a visitors' centre noted for its sea bathing, which was regarded as a health-giving pursuit for much of the eighteenth century. Early in the nineteenth century the spa – or 'spaw' as it was called locally – was redeveloped by the Cliff Bridge Company and in 1826 it was re-opened. Scarborough quickly became a fashionable resort for Victorian England; by 1867 it could describe itself proudly as "Queen of the Watering Places".

By the 1850s, then, hotels, lodging houses, inns and the catering trade, not to mention medicine and entertainment, had, with shipbuilding, generated reliable employment for Scarborough's inhabitants for well over a century. Reflecting this prosperity, the population grew from about 6,000 in the mid eighteenth century to 13,000 in the mid nineteenth and over 33,000 by that century's end. The boom was boosted by the arrival of the railway in 1845, opening new markets to the expanding fishing industry and enabling it to exploit more effectively Scarborough's proximity to the abundant fishing grounds of the North Sea's Dogger Bank. The railway also transformed Scarborough from a rather select watering place for the gentry to a mass holiday resort. As happened in many parts of Victorian Britain, the arrival of the railway also initiated a spate of urban renewal, and much was done to improve the public buildings, the housing and the infra-structure of the town in the 1850s.

Not everyone, however, shared in this economic abundance. The shipbuilding industry went into decline as the century progressed and by 1860 had all but vanished: two small yards remained active, constructing fishing yawls.

Thomas Postgate's trade, joinery, which must have relied considerably on shipbuilding, would have been contracting in the 1830s. He had a large family, and it is reasonable to guess that times were not easy for them. This is probably why the young John Postgate, displaying his own distinctive personality at an early age, left home voluntarily, obtaining at the age of eleven employment as a apprentice to a grocer and wine merchant. His pay was 3/6d (17½ p) a week, not ungenerous for the time. Gradually he became aware of adulteration practices such as those described in the first chapter, and after three years he had become so disgusted with the trade that he resolved to quit.

He had taught himself a little chemistry and, learning in the spring of 1834 that a partnership of Scarborough surgeons was seeking an assistant, he applied for the post. He was successful. He took a considerable cut in pay, to a miserable 2/6d (12½ p) a week, but his employers, Mr Travis and Mr Dunn, were soon highly impressed by his diligence as a dispenser, and advised him to enter the medical profession. He was articled to their firm for five years, which gave him security, and he set about the first step, the study of pharmacy, with enthusiasm. He not only dedicated his ordinary leisure to study, he would also rise at five o'clock in the morning to get in some extra reading before work. His first hurdle would be an examination at Apothecaries' Hall. Simultaneously he had to teach himself Latin, in those days a requirement for a medical career, and was soon reading Eutropius and Caesar's *De Bello Gallico*. His energy and dedication were impressive. He also continued chemistry, improved his general knowledge, and became fascinated by botany. In the summer months he would rise even earlier, at three or four in the morning, to seek specimens of wild plants in the neighbourhood and countryside. He made an almost complete collection of the wild plants of the locality, and preserved his specimens in a herbarium which he still possessed, with pride, in 1880; in 1837 the *Yorkshire Magazine* published a paper by him, a 17-year old, on "Rare Plants and their Properties" [2.4]. One wonders whether he had any time to visit his parents and siblings during this period.

In 1839 he completed his apprenticeship and the firm took him on as an assistant. This change of status and pay enabled him to save money, intended at some future date to pay for lectures, provided he could get work within reach of a medical school. Five years later, in 1844*, he had sufficient saved up and, recommended by Travis and Dunn, he obtained a position as Assistant Apothecary to the public dispensary at Leeds, which was associated with the Leeds School of Medicine. This post carried board and lodging and a stipend of £10 a year, and time off had been arranged for him to attend lectures within the School. There he remained for three years. There was considerable pressure of work in the dispensary, and he found many of the drugs to be impure; nevertheless, he distinguished himself academically in the Medical School and obtained 'first medals' for chemistry, materia medica and botany.

In July of 1847* he went to London to be examined at the Society of Apothecaries, and passed with flying colours: the Court of Examiners complimented him both on his Latin and on his professional ability. Duly he received his licence to practice, and he obtained a post as an assistant in a large medical practice in East London. He also registered himself as a student in surgery at the London Hospital and its Medical College.

To a bright and inquisitive young man from Yorkshire, even one forewarned by a taste of urban life in Leeds, London in the 1840s must have come as something of a shock. As Henry Mayhew recorded so vividly [2.5], the metropolis was overcrowded, dirty, noisy, smelly and often dangerous. The population had swelled from over 700 000 in 1800 to over 2 million, an increase accommodated largely by crowding and expanding the existing housing. The streets were a *mêlée* of costermongers and street traders, beggars and petty thieves, street urchins, clerks and messengers, pimps and prostitutes, an amorphous population going about its regular business among stalls, handcarts,

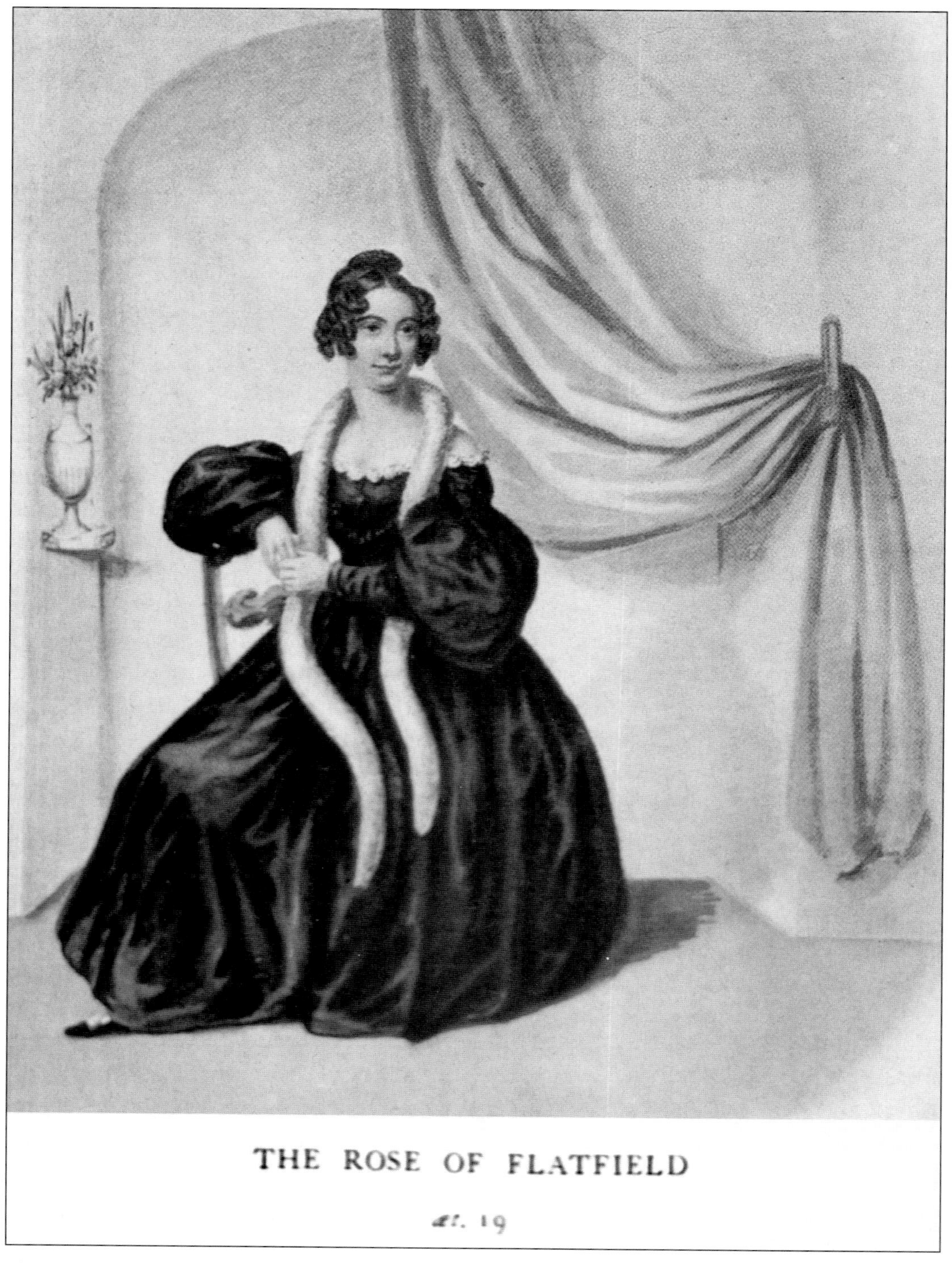

A presumptive likeness of Mary Ann Horwood aged 19. From Isabella Postgate's A Trilogy of Victorian Saints *[reference 2.7]*

horses and carriages. Nowhere in Europe was the gap between rich and poor more blatant.

Much of East London already consisted of slum 'rookeries'. Deformities and disease were rife; parasitism, exploitation and crime were rampant. Like many another Victorian of goodwill, Postgate was appalled. Everywhere he looked, ordinary people were being exploited. Apart from theft and low wages, such food as they could afford was unreliable and adulterated, as he had learned in Scarborough. And his experience as a dispenser had now taught him that medicines and drugs were flagrantly adulterated, too. And doubtless he had come across the strongly reformist periodical for the medical profession, *The Lancet*, which had come into being in 1823; it had exposed the use of potentially poisonous adulterants in the confectionery trade, and was busily advocating proper sanitation and public health measures. A spirit of reform was in the air – but before he could do anything constructive about it himself, he had to become qualified.

After the seemingly short period of a year he was able to pass his examination for the Royal College of Surgeons and became a Member of that body in July of 1848*.

As an MRCS he was fully qualified professionally. He had remained in touch with his erstwhile employers, and Mr Dunn recommended him for a position in Sherburn, a dozen miles South East of Scarborough in Yorkshire, under the auspices of William Henry, 7th Viscount Downe, head of the Dawnay family. They owned the substantial Wykeham Estate at Wykeham. However, it is unlikely that a position tied to nobility would have suited a determined, self-made young doctor with a developing sense of public duty. He declined the offer and joined a surgical practice in Kilham, some 17 miles due South of Scarborough. Here he found time to help establish a library and literary institution, where he gave lectures in chemistry and botany. He was already displaying the public-spirited outlook which came to dominate his life.

Kilham was, and still is, a small country town, a centre for a small rural population. To set up an institute at all in such a community during the late 1840s was an innovative measure. Its Institute would have been a rural forerunner of the successful Working Men's Institutes and Clubs which were founded in the 1850s and '60s in the larger towns and cities by the Reverend

---

*These years differ from those in a brief contemporary biography [2.6], which quotes years that are inconsistent with its own text, at least one being an evident misprint. Some of these mistakes were perpetuated in certain obituary notices and also in his entry in the Dictionary of National Biography of 1909 [2.7]. The years given above are more plausible in the light of the surrounding events of his life.

Henry Solly. A one-time Chartist, Solly canvassed subscriptions from business men and aristocrats to finance a network of clubs (the 'Working Men's Club and Institute Union') for the education and relaxation of the working classes. Solly was an enthusiast, and was very effective at raising support for his clubs and institutes; his first institute was established in 1852, later than the Kilham Institute, and his movement did not become widespread for another decade, after 1862. (He also had the austerity typical of a romantic radical: the clubs, to which the users were expected to subscribe, were to be teetotal, non-smoking communities dedicated to reading, rest and self-improvement. In fact they were notably under-subscribed in their early days and relied almost wholly on upper- and middle-class subsidies for finance. Indeed, among their supporters was Queen Victoria, who presented the Union with a consignment of autographed copies of *The Early Years Of The Prince Consort.*) Despite their financial fragility the Institutes and Clubs flourished and proved to be durable, and some 2,400 exist to this day. In accordance with Solly's vision they are now largely self-financing, but their teetotal character was soon abandoned – indeed, some claim that their relatively cheap beer has been the main reason for their durability – and during the twentieth century most of their educational function became displaced by the provision of entertainment. Today they are popular social clubs, some distinctly wealthy, but their working-class roots are far from forgotten.

The Kilham Institute, located next to a Primitive Chapel close to the school, survived into the mid twentieth century but today its site is occupied by a private bungalow. John Postgate's services to the community were recognized in September of 1849 when he was presented with a "testimonial", raised by public subscription. (A testimonial, in this usage, was a gift, inscribed or appropriately certificated, presented as a mark of appreciation; it was often accompanied by residual money from the subscription.)

About six miles further South from Kilham lay the market town of Driffield. Here one Joshua Horwood RN (b.1781) was a general practitioner, a highly respected surgeon who had served under Lord Nelson on the *Prince* at the Battle of Trafalgar and received the Trafalgar Medal. He died in 1850 and John Postgate took over his practice. This Joshua Horwood was the son of an earlier Joshua (b.1751) by his wife Ann Langdale; the earlier Joshua's father, David Horwood, had circumnavigated the globe with Captain Cook. Joshua of Driffield married Hariett Foord and sired three children, Mary Ann (b.1815), Joshua (b.1817) and Henery, who died young.

A portrait of Mary Ann, seemingly a watercolour painted when she was nineteen years old, forms the frontispiece of a trio of biographical essays (see pp.65 to 66) published by her daughter Isabella [2.8]: in Mary Ann, we see a beautiful Victorian maiden, with an intelligent and refined expression. She was well-educated and cultured, and as a young woman she wrote poetry and had literary aspirations. Her personal writing album, which Isabella still possessed in 1930, indicated that she was much sought after by young men. Yet she had chosen none of them, and was a 35-year-old spinster when John Postgate arrived in Driffield. Remarkably soon, in May of 1851, she and Postgate were married at Aston church in Birmingham – a "hasty and ill-advised" union according to Isabella – and, after a honeymoon tour, Postgate having quit the Driffield practice about this time, they settled in Birmingham, where he set himself up as a general practitioner. There they remained for the rest of their lives.

Chapter 3

BIRMINGHAM

Birmingham in the first couple of decades of the nineteenth century was a handsome, spacious country town, with elegant houses and gardens and the river Rea as its axis. But all over England the migration of population from the countryside to towns was bringing with it poverty, disease, squalour and overcrowding. To peasants and labourers abandoning the countryside, the attractions of urban life were tremendous: reasonably well-paid jobs in the rapidly expanding industries and services, new uses for old skills in tool-making, construction and transport, scope for acquiring new skills, and all sorts of entrepreneurial opportunities – plus an exciting environment with shops and entertainments. Undoubtedly many benefitted, but a great many more did not. Capitalism was growing in a succession of booms and slumps, and with each slump thousands upon thousands lost their jobs. In possibly the worst slump of that era, around 1842, up to four fifths of the work-force from certain Midlands industries joined the ranks of the unemployed. Meanwhile housing in cities had in no way kept up with the inward migration, and whole areas became squalid and overcrowded ghettos, fraught with poverty, malnutrition and disease, especially in London.

Existing ways of relieving poverty could not cope, and in 1834 Parliament had set up a Royal Commission on Reform of the Poor Law, with physician Edwin (later Sir Edwin) Chadwick as its Secretary. Chadwick's reports to the Commission entitled *The Sanitary Condition of the Labouring Population* (1832) and *The Health of Towns* (1834) were momentous documents which shocked the nation and led ultimately to Parliament's passing the Public Health Act of 1848. But the immediate reforms which Chadwick, through his Commission, prescribed, and which were embodied in the New Poor Law of 1834, though well-intentioned, were a disaster [3.1].

By 1851, when the Postgates moved into their house at 80 Belmont Row, parts of Birmingham were already slums, poverty-stricken and overcrowded. Birmingham's population was expanding remorselessly and would rise by a half again over the next twenty years – excluding those who lived outside its municipal boundaries. The civic situation was not so dire as in London, but it had become sufficiently threatening for the Public Health Board (a Local Government body established under the Public Health Act of 1848 [3.2]) to commission an enquiry. Their inspector, Mr Robert Rawlinson, reported in

1849 that many of Birmingham's attractive houses had been built round closed and dark courts, and that these had become "foul and foetid" [3.3]. They had been "ill-built", were undrained and lacked proper sanitation, their cellars often half full of water. Insanitary liquid accumulated in their courtyards and overflowed into the roads, where people would use bricks as stepping stones. Wells were contaminated, yielding water "green as a leek". The River Rea was obstructed with debris and was covered with "a thick scum of decomposing matter". The worst areas had become "the haunts of vice, the resorts of thieves". Fevers and typhus were common, though Birmingham had so far escaped cholera epidemics such as had recently afflicted Liverpool and Manchester.

Rawlinson recommended drastic action, including slum clearance, proper drainage, proper water supplies and sewerage, but for several reasons the Town Council failed to act decisively. For one thing, it resented the interference by Government in municipal affairs; for another, the Council shared responsibility for the infrastructure of Birmingham – paving, cleaning, lighting, sanitation etc – with no fewer than seven other Boards, an administrative complexity which led to gross inefficiency and conflicts of planning; and again, monuments, parks and civic ceremony were more to its taste than costly urban renewal. The administrative problem was eased in 1851 when an Act of Parliament enabled the Town Council to acquire overall responsibility for public health from the various boards but, despite local pressure, turbulence at Council meetings, even angry resignations of Councillors, little happened until about 1857, when some remedial action was put in hand. Indeed, it was not until the 1860s that serious action was taken, as the arrival of the railway catalysed "the first great wave of slum clearance in Birmingham" [3.4], that of the 1860s and '70s. Then massive rebuilding was undertaken, the courts and elegant gardens disappeared and the transformation of Birmingham into a city began. Even so, it required the Public Health Act of 1872 to induce the Town Council to take sewerage and water seriously in hand, and even at that date squalid slum areas were still abundant in the New Street area.

Not surprisingly, the insanitary state of Birmingham was an early public issue to engage Postgate's attention, once he had established his practice at Belmont Row. He followed the local political arguments and protests closely and in 1852 added his own contribution in the form of a pamphlet, published at his own expense from Belmont Row, entitled "The Sanatary Aspect of Birmingham and Suggestions for its Improvement" [3.5].

He was clearly impatient with those who grumbled or protested but did nothing constructive. His pamphlet's object was "...not to investigate minutely or utter querulous complaints of admitted ills, but to suggest a remedy..." Nevertheless, he had to introduce his pamphlet with some account of the actual

THE

SANATARY ASPECT

OF

BIRMINGHAM,

AND

SUGGESTIONS FOR ITS IMPROVEMENT.

BY JOHN POSTGATE, M.R.C.S.

&c., &c., &c.

BIRMINGHAM:

THOMAS RAGG, 90, HIGH STREET.

1852.

Preface.

The object of the following remarks is not to investigate minutely or utter querulous complaints of admitted ills, but to suggest a remedy, and by the proposed Birmingham Sanatary Society, to enforce existant powers, and obtain others if those are inefficient.

The Author's intention is well meant, and candidly stated. He hopes the proposition will be received in the same spirit; and fairly discussed.

It will afford him pleasure to communicate with any gentleman desirous of forwarding these views either personally at his residence, or by letter.

80, Belmont Row, Birmingham,
January, 1852.

Cover page and Preface of John Postgate's first pamphlet.

problem, and he did so with an impressive combination of indignation and astonishment. Efforts, he acknowledged, were being made to keep the "better class of streets" (Islington, Broad Street, Paradise Street, New Street, High Street, Dale End and Coleshill Street [3.6]), and some of their side streets, clean and regularly swept. But in others, including his own Belmont Row, dirt from the gutters had been brushed into numerous heaps and left, obstructing drainage, generating puddles and rendering the street "nearly impassable". The heaps were removed only when "noxious gases generated during putrefaction had escaped and poisoned the air" – or rain had washed the debris back into the gutters. But some mess clearly remained: Great Barr Street [3.6], he observed, had become as black and rutty as an unmended road on the moors. Refuse and open sewers "contaminating the air by noisome effluvia and *inviting* epidemic diseases, fevers &c., are a blot and a disgrace to a large town abounding in wealth and intelligence...," he wrote.

More alarming to his readers would have been his evocative remarks on the sanitary consequences of urban graveyards, a topic of the day which had been raised earlier by a Mr Walker (possibly Joseph Walker, a contemporary Birmingham magistrate with an interest in municipal matters):

> "Interment in towns!", Postgate wrote, "what is it but allowing decomposing flesh to poison the air we breathe; Ay! and further, when a shower descends to mix the water we drink with the fluid of dead bodies!... Let anyone observe our elevated Church Yards, crowded with dead, deposited in sand and gravel, through which the rain freely passes, and let him shew, if he can, that part of this water does not mix with the spring which supplies the well with the water he drinks. Close, then, all your burial grounds in town, – to remain monuments of bygone ignorance, and let your dead be interred away from the haunts of the living, – where in some sylvan scene the tear of grief may fall and the sigh escape undisturbed by a busy throng."

The main thrust of his pamphlet, however, concerned air quality (a problem which is still with us a century and a half later, albeit in a new form). He urged the acquisition of a large private park at Aston for public use, parks being "the lungs of large places", and devoted much of his space to the smoke and fumes which plagued Birmingham at that time. Although the town had not yet felt the full impact of the industrial revolution, smoke pollution had become so bad that the Council had appointed a special inspector in 1844 to patrol and restrict emissions from the 176 chimneys serving coal-fired steam engines, furnaces and boilers located within the town. But his efforts were largely ineffectual: by 1851 some 280 chimneys were now discharging such smoke, often dense and black, often for much of the day, supplementing smoke from domestic coal-burning grates. Yet, Postgate wrote, relatively cheap smoke-consuming equipment was commercially available to industry, and actually allowed economies in fuel consumption.

A problem for Postgate was that there was no firm medical evidence, at that time, that smoke was harmful, and he had to turn to polemic. But his argument gives an insight on ordinary living in 1850s Birmingham:

> "It is stated, and frequently too, by persons who cannot see their real interest, that, contrary to every-day experience, smoke is not injurious to health. But I am not writing medically, and will therefore merely ask those individuals, How it happens that we are obliged every morning to make a short cough or effort to remove a tenacious mass of soot and mucus? Is it natural to expectorate this? Is the irritation that smoke produces in the lungs and air passages, where there is a tendency to disease[,] likely to diminish or

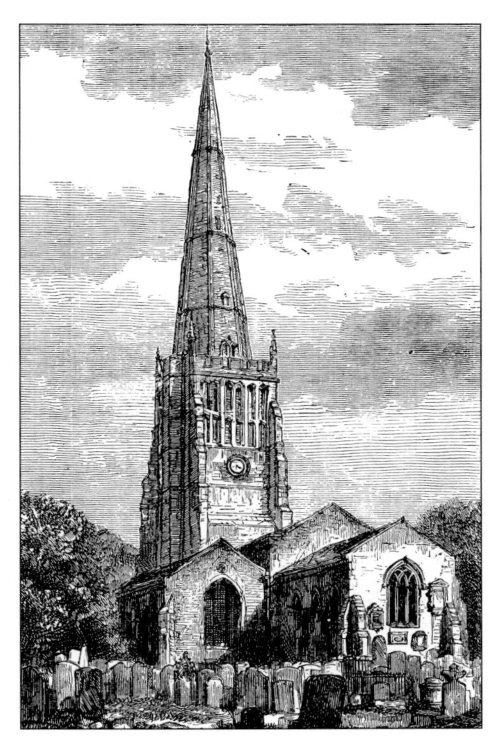

Aston Church

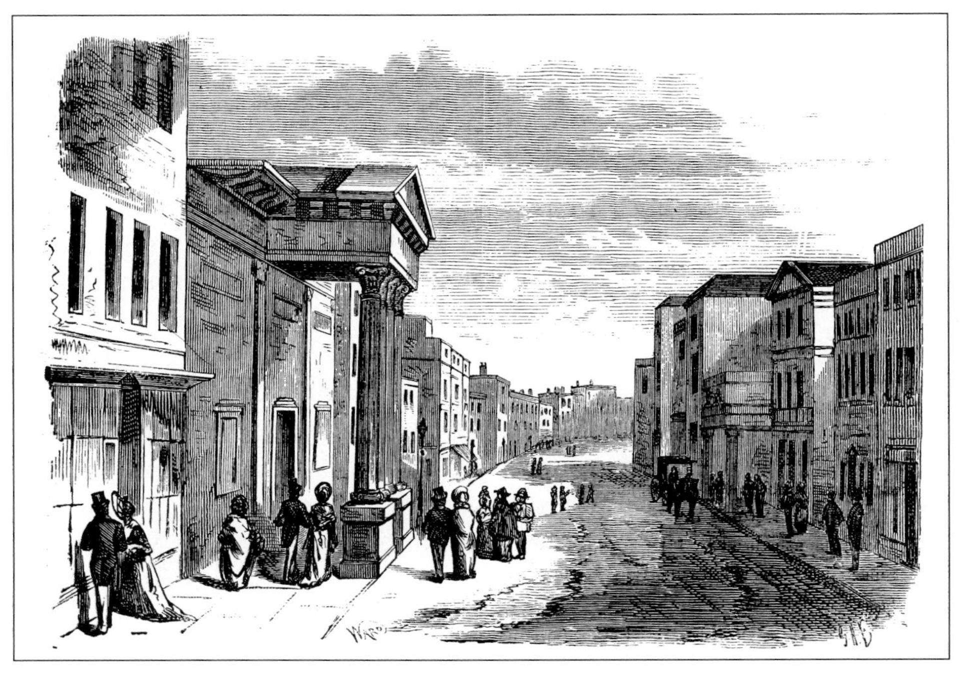

Old view of the top of New Street, showing the Society of Artists' Rooms.

> increase it? If dense smoke is not injurious, why do those persons who produce it, retreat to their villas and country seats, miles from its influence? ..."

His pamphlet concluded with his own proposal: that a "Birmingham Sanatary Society" be formed with the objective of studying the health of operatives in the context of their employment, to consider the effects of local conditions on epidemics of disease, to enforce the existing law on sanitary matters, to report to and advise the Town Council and, if necessary, to lobby for further powers from Government.

Though this proposal amounted, in effect, to setting up a forward-looking local programme of field research in social medicine, it was not radical and need not have been costly. The necessary legislation already existed, empowering the Town Council to enforce control of emissions, to designate park land, to relocate graveyards, to cope with sewage, water pollution and so on. And such a 'Society', to include a committee, an inspector, a solicitor and a secretary, would not be an untoward charge on the rates. However, a Town Council that had so recently escaped from the deadlocks and obstructions generated by a multitude of Municipal Boards was unlikely to welcome a new semi-autonomous advisory body. It is hardly surprising that no such Society was formed. Moreover, as B T Davis pointed out [3.7], though Postgate was not the sort of man to be deterred by irresolution on the Council's part, his own determination to push the matter ahead was moderated by other events in his professional career. But in the broader context of the reforms being demanded in Birmingham, his pamphlet introduced new ideas and straight thinking. For Postgate himself, it indicated that he had understood a simple but important fact of politics: that to make a serious contribution to a social issue you must not only delineate that issue evocatively, you must also prescribe to your politicians, in as much detail as possible, their most plausible way of taking action. It was an understanding that would inform his later, and more successful, efforts to bring about the control by Government of adulteration of food and drugs.

An immediate distraction, which would certainly have demanded a great deal of Postgate's attention, was the beginning of his academic career, which he would subsequently pursue in parallel with his ordinary medical practice. A new medical school, Sydenham College, was set up in 1851, an off-shoot of Birmingham's General Hospital and a rival to Queen's College Medical School [3.8]. In 1852, after only a year in local practice, John Postgate was appointed its demonstrator of anatomy and lecturer on surgical and descriptive anatomy, a position he held until early 1855, when he became lecturer on medical jurisprudence. He had also been continuing his own studies and, after passing the necessary examinations, he was admitted a Fellow of the Royal College of Surgeons on May 11, 1854.

He was not distracted from reformist activity for long, however. Sanitation and public health were, in the 1850s, very live issues among people of goodwill; dear to the heart of the writer Charles Kingsley, for example, who wrote about and lectured on them. Perhaps because many people of influence had the cause of sanitation and public health well in hand, Postgate turned his attention to the scandals of which he had had direct professional experience, the adulteration of food and of drugs.

The growth of urban populations in the early decades of the nineteenth century had not only had dire social consequences in terms of poverty and overcrowding, it had also led to radical changes in the distribution of food. In the past, rural communities had for the most part consumed food produced at home, or bought from neighbours, perhaps by way of small local markets. The smaller towns had been largely provisioned from the surrounding countryside, country-folk bringing in their produce on regular market days. Of course, in towns there had always been shops which sold specialised products, and goods which came from afar such as sugar and tea, and with the growth of cities the population became increasingly dependent on such professional retailers: butchers, bakers, grocers, as well as the more specialised food and drink shops, themselves dependent on wholesalers and from specialised markets offering meat, vegetables and so on. The transition to a society depending largely on a professional food trade was given added impetus by the arrival of the railways, which enabled the fast transport of perishables such as fish from the coast, and of imported materials from London and other ports. In effect, the marketing of food was shifting from a local or regional basis to a national one, presaging the early twentieth-century pre-supermarket pattern in which locally-produced food would become an urban rarity. This was no great loss to the new urban citizens, for rural nutrition had long been sparse and monotonous [3.9], and on the positive side there were substantial benefits in terms of the choices available, even to those on modest incomes, and access to commodities such as tea and spices that were once luxuries of the aristocracy. That was true for those who could pay; yet, especially during the 1840s, many lived on the poverty line and could only afford scraps and left-overs. More fortunate people were shocked at the near-starvation to be seen on the streets of big cities, where inadequate diets might be supplemented by scavenged rancid, wilted, rotting or simply dirty foodstuffs. Typical of such charitable concern, the famous chef Alexis Soyer instigated soup kitchens, financed by public subscription, in the streets of London and Dublin when, in 1847, shortages of potatoes and flour had made conditions especially arduous [3.10].

The sometimes huge populations of unemployed, especially in times of slump, kept the prices of really cheap food down. However, with the changes in food distribution had come a concomitant increase in the scope for adulteration and fraud, from which the poor and their dependents were likely to suffer most, for they could afford only the very cheapest and could not be selective. In the words of Friedrich Engels, writing in 1845:

> "... the poor, the working people, to whom a couple of farthings are important, who must buy things with little money, who cannot afford to inquire too closely into the quality of their purchase, and cannot do so in any case because they have no opportunity of cultivating their taste – to their share fall all the adulterated, poisoned provisions." [3.11]

The scandal of adulteration and its evil consequences in terms of health, especially among the poor, were entirely familiar to John Postgate. However, there were many ills in early Victorian society to command the attention of one of reforming disposition: it was a case which arose in his own practice that provoked him into action. One of his patients, a woman, suffered an alarming attack of diarrhoea and vomiting after drinking coffee. He examined the coffee and it proved to contain not only chicory, but also some noxious black substance to which he attributed its toxicity (though he did not in fact identify it).

It was as a direct result of this experience that he embarked upon a public campaign against the scandal which obsessed him for the rest of his life.

Chapter 4

A CAMPAIGN BEGINS

The scandal of food adulteration in Britain had been brought into the public eye in 1820, with the publication of the first extensive account of the subject: F C Accum's *A Treatise on Adulterations of Food and Culinary Poisons* [4.1]. Accum (1769-1838) was a chemist and an engineer. He was born in Germany and in 1793 came to Britain, where he had an impressive career which included lecturing on chemistry and physics and writing books on general chemistry (including a collection of "entertaining" chemistry experiments for boys). He also wrote on coal gas, mineralogy, crystallography, and on chemistry as applied to building materials, to food, to brewing, to baking and to wine-making. A chemical polymath, he is widely known among civil engineers as one of the instigators of the use of coal gas for street lighting in British towns, in particular when he was working for the newly-formed Gas, Light and Coke Company of London after 1810. In 1801 he had been made 'Assistant Chemical Operator' at the Royal Institution in London, a prestigious appointment, and he became a popular public figure for his writings and lectures on chemistry. He resigned from the Institution in 1803 to teach and lecture at his own private college; his career progressed to include a Chair at the Surrey Institution. Late in 1820, however, his brilliant career in Britain was brought to an abrupt stop: he was charged with 'robbery'. The crime seems to have been defacement of books in the library of the Royal Institution, a charge of removing pages having been dismissed at trial. A proud and sensitive personality, he not unreasonably returned to Germany where, within a couple of years, he became a Professor at Berlin's Technical Institute. He remained there for the rest of his life [4.2].

When first published, Accum's treatise made a great impression on the establishment and the general public, and it went into several editions, including imprints in Germany and the USA. But it generated considerable antagonism among commercial interests, and its popular nature and lack of quantitative detail laid it open to doubts about the actual extent of the adulterative practices it claimed to expose. These criticisms, together with the taint of scandal associated with its author's trial, enabled his opponents to undermine confidence in the work, and by 1824 it was widely regarded as exaggerated [4.3]. It was not exaggerated, but though the evil of food adulteration was aired in specialised texts during the 1840s [4.4], it was a series of articles in *The Lancet* which brought adulteration into the public arena again. Primarily responsible for *The Lancet*'s campaign was its editor, Dr Thomas Wakley (1795-1862). He was another remarkable man [4.5]. He had founded *The Lancet* in 1823 (it is still one of the most widely-read British medical journals) and remained its editor for life. In addition he became member of Parliament for Finsbury, North London, in 1835, and represented that constituency until an election in 1852, when he retired from parliament voluntarily. He was a popular M.P. because of his support for reformist and liberal causes, especially those bearing upon public health. He was also elected Coroner for West Middlesex, in which capacity he showed such concern for the treatment of paupers that he became known as 'The Radical Coroner'. A famous episode was the dreadful affair of Thomas Austin, a resident of the Hendon workhouse, who, in 1839, fell into the laundry 'copper' and was scalded to death. The workhouse authorities quietly buried him and did not notify his death to the coroner. Wakley got to hear of it and was incensed; he sought an exhumation, which was refused, and insisted upon an inquest which, after some opposition, was held. The cause of death was clear, but Wakley added a rider to the effect that the master of the workhouse had been guilty of contributory negligence in not providing a protective railing round the copper. The master commented resentfully:

> "The jury have found a verdict, but have not identified the body."

To which Wakley made a reply for which he became celebrated:

> "If this is not the body of the man who was killed in your vat, pray, Sir, how many paupers have you boiled?"

Under Wakley's editorship *The Lancet* was a crusading, reforming periodical, concerned with improving the quality of medicine as generally practised and with exposing inefficiency and nepotism in hospitals. It reported medical lectures and published case reports from which all could learn, and very soon it was exposing quackery and fraud. It took up the blatantly obvious need for public-health measures in many aspects of mid-century life and was much preoccupied with sanitation and hygiene. As a professional doctor, Postgate would have been well aware of it and its campaigns.

Shortly after taking his seat in parliament in 1835, Wakley became concerned about the quality of foodstuffs as they were marketed to the general public. He would have known of, and probably read, Accum's pioneering treatise, and in 1830 he had asked Dr William (later Sir William) Brooks O'Shaughnessy to analyse samples of confectionery, the results of which he published under the title *Poisoned confectionery* in *The Lancet* next year [4.6]. O'Shaughnessy had found lead, copper and mercury derivatives in various samples of sugar confectionery, all toxic additives, and also gamboge, a powerful purgative of vegetable origin. They had been added as colouring agents. In his article he had also drawn attention to the presence of such poisons on sweet wrappers, which young children were likely to suck or lick. O'Shaughnessy had presented his data to the then Home Secretary, but no action had followed. In 1836-37 Wakley had also arranged for some analyses of foodstuffs by T H Henry FRS, but he had not felt able to initiate sustained pressure for remedial legislation for many years, partly because of other activities, partly because, Accum's work being in disrepute, a new and substantial body of well-documented evidence on the subject was needed. Although adulteration was widely known to be on the increase, hard evidence describing the then current situation was scarce.

It is likely that a lecture to the Botanical Society of London in 1850, given by physician and microscopist Arthur Hill Hassall, alerted Wakley that the time for action had come.

Dr. Hassall had sent Wakley a copy of his paper. He was yet another impressive Victorian polymath [4.7]. Trained as a surgeon, then becoming a physician and lecturer at the Royal Free Hospital in London, he combined general practice with investigations in zoology, botany, anatomy and public health. Using mainly the microscope, he published important studies of zoophytes (aquatic animals which resemble plants, such as the coelenterates) and of aquatic algae; he established the role of fungi in the rotting of fruit and vegetables; his published description of Thames water, the principal source of drinking water for the whole metropolis, in the words of his biographer, makes the flesh creep [4.8]:

> "Let the observer walk along the banks of the river for a short distance and the following will, in most instances, be the result of his observations:
> "in one spot he will notice the carcasses of dead animals, rotting, festering, swarming with flies and maggots, and from which a pestilential odour proceeds, ... in another he will see a variety of refuse born along by the lazy current of the stream – decaying vegetables, the leaves and stalks of cabbages, grass from a new-mown lawn, excrement ... he will perceive some sewer, discharging its corrupt and filthy contents ...
> "... If [in the shallows] he plunges his hand into the water, he will bring up a dirty, slimy mass..."

Illustrated in colour, with depictions of the aquatic microflora, Hassall's report caused public outcry; a parliamentary Committee of Enquiry was set up, to which he gave evidence, and, in 1852, an Act was passed requiring the London water companies to take water only from above Teddington Lock.

He made numerous contributions to general medicine; he certainly saw

THE *LANCET'S* DETECTIVE FORCE.

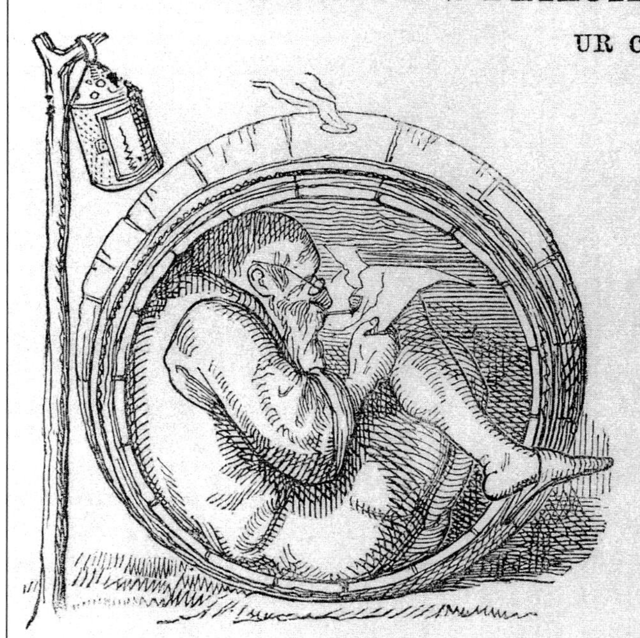

UR contemporary the *Lancet* has conferred a great boon on the public by establishing a new order of constabulary, which may be called the Scientific Detective Police. The function of these Detectives is to investigate and expose the fraudulent adulteration of articles of food practised by a set of scoundrels under the names of grocers and other tradesmen. In his researches into this rascality, the *Lancet's* policeman is assisted by a microscope, which, in throwing light on the fraud in question, exerts a power far superior to that of the common bull's eye. By the help of this instrument, an immense quantity of villanous stuff has been discovered in coffee, arrowroot, and other substances sold for nutriment, and, some of them, "particularly recommended to invalids." The *Lancet* seconds the exertions of its intelligent officer by spiritedly publishing the addresses of the rogues at whose swindling establishments the samples of rubbish were purchased. If any of the knaves thus pilloried in the *Lancet*, abetted by a disreputable attorney and a dishonest barrister, endeavour to avenge themselves through the technicalities of the law, *Punch* hopes they will meet with twelve true men in the jury-box who will scout both them and their legal accomplices out of court.

Punch*'s view of* The Lancet*'s Analytical Sanitary Commission, from an issue of February, 1851, p65.*

cholera vibrios in the stools of cholera victims during London's epidemic of 1854, though neither he nor anyone else was yet convinced that they were the actual pathogen; he described the morphology of the cells of the thymus gland; he founded a tuberculosis sanatorium in the Isle of Wight. In the mid 1860s his health began to break down and in due course he retired to San Remo, where he died.

In almost all these contexts, Hassall's major research tool had been the microscope. As far as his seminal work on the adulteration of coffee was concerned, he had had the elegantly simple idea of inspecting coffee and possible adulterants under the microscope, and observed that their microstructure was sufficiently well preserved after roasting for inspection to be an adequate check for adulteration. In his lecture he reported that he had examined 34 samples of ground coffee, mostly of ostensibly high quality, and identified adulterants including chicory, roasted corn, roasted peas, potato flour or bean flour in 31. On other occasions he found crushed mangel-wurzel and pounded acorns in coffee.

Hassall was by no means the first scientist to use microscopy for the identification of materials. In 1840, Jonathan Pereira of the newly-formed Pharmaceutical Society had used it to check on types of starch and others had used it to detect adulteration of coffee and tea. But Hassall was the first to exploit it systematically and quantitatively, examining many samples and recording the numerical extent of adulteration. Wakley was impressed by the power of microscopy in this context and decided that he could now, in the 1850s, add food adulteration to *The Lancet*'s several reformist causes. Hassall became an indispensable colleague in this campaign; Wakley commissioned him, paying for his materials plus a salary, to examine a variety of foods on behalf of *The Lancet*, and in 1851, the year in which Postgate moved to Birmingham, *The Lancet* published the first of a series of articles exposing food adulteration.

That article announced the setting up of the *The Lancet*'s "Analytical Sanitary Commission" the objective of which was expressed so:

> "We propose, then, for the public benefit to institute an extensive and somewhat vigorous series of investigations into the present condition of the various articles of diet supplied to the inhabitants of this great metropolis and its vicinity, and probably the inquiries will be extended to some of our distant cities and towns."[4.9].

'Vigorous' meant that the Commission would seek its own samples, do its own analyses, chemical and microscopical, and would report regularly, naming names where appropriate. The Analytical Sanitary Commission in fact comprised Wakley and O'Shaughnessy [4.10], neither of whom did actual tests, and Hassall, working with great enthusiasm. Hassall sometimes sub-contracted tests, in particular to Dr Henry Letheby [4.11], who was a more experienced analytical chemist (later Medical Officer of Health for the City of London); he also used other analysts infrequently, generally to substantiate findings when his own might have been disputed. Hassall did not restrict his studies simply to adulteration; he investigated other kinds of fraud as well, such as the substitution of cheap sardines or spratts, salted and dyed, for the more expensive anchovies.

The Commission's reports continued to be published for four years, weekly at first, then fortnightly. In addition to coffee, Hassall examined tea, sugar (in which he saw mites among other contaminants), arrowroot, London water, chicory, mustard, bread, cocoa, farinaceous foods and sixteen other ordinary items of food, as well as opium and tobacco. He uncovered some horrifying practices: alum in all of 49 samples of bread; red lead (an oxide of lead) in cayenne pepper; lead chromate, red lead, copper arsenide or white lead (hydrated lead carbonate), among other unpleasant or dangerous substances, used to colour sweetmeats. All these additives were known to be toxic in the 1850s, the lead and copper salts especially so. As it had threatened to do, *The Lancet* did include the names and addresses of manufacturers and tradesmen whom the Commission had caught out, which meant that Wakley, as its editor, was taking a considerable risk with the libel laws. *The Lancet*'s reports were diligently reported by the wider press and made an enormous impression on the general public. They even featured in *Punch*: in 1851 it made typical serio-comic play about "the horrid adulterations of tea", maintaining that their exposure had led to an abrupt upsurge in cognac consumption in the metropolis. It also argued that Her Majesty's Customs Officials would be better occupied watching out for contaminated imports than harassing private travellers [4.13]. But predictably *The Lancet* became very unpopular with the grocery trade.

Hassall conducted his most intensive research into adulteration during some five years between 1849 and 1854, scaling it down thereafter as he turned to other interests, though he did not discontinue it altogether. He collated and extended his work for *The Lancet* for publication as a book [4.12]. The body of that work proved to be extremely important as far as ultimate legislation was concerned and, together with his work on water purity and cholera, it made him a household name: he (and Letheby) even achieved a mention in Charles Kingsley's *The Water-Babies* [4.14] a popular moral fantasy for children. But as many a social activist has found, his fame also generated abuse and criticism. This was especially so among tradesmen. And he sometimes inspired jealousy and annoyance among his scientific peers, some of whom, while they may not have disagreed with his objectives in principle, believed their contributions had been slighted, or that he overstated his case. For though he was a courteous man, he seems to have been a domineering figure. He clashed with Letheby, several of his scientific peers refused to support a testimonial dinner which was planned for him in 1855 (and which took place nevertheless [4.15]), and even his relations with Wakley became briefly soured. Such matters will be discussed further in Chapter 8.

It was not until 1857 that Wakley and Hassall extended their investigation outside London, examining samples from four provincial towns, Birmingham, Leeds, Liverpool and Manchester. In Birmingham, at least, the ground had been prepared; by 1854 John Postgate would have known all about *The Lancet*'s campaign, and the abuses of foodstuffs thereby exposed were familiar to him from his days as a grocer's apprentice. He also discovered illnesses among his own patients which could be assigned to poisons in food or drink. But there is no evidence that he had any direct contact with *The Lancet*'s 'Commission'; he seems to have embarked upon his own campaign independently.

Wakley and Hassell were relying mainly upon publicity for effect. It would not only shame offending grocers and bring them into public disrepute, it would also hit them in the pockets, as it were. At the same time it would bring the scandalous situation to the attention of the wider public, as well as local and national authorities. The pair were successful: the daily press approvingly printed long excerpts from *The Lancet*'s articles. The furore generated by *The Lancet*'s Commission had been such that the Chancellor of the Exchequer (Sir Charles Wood) was moved to defend the addition of chicory to coffee in his budget speech for 1851. (Its addition had been approved by the Treasury as a harmless, even beneficial, way of making coffee cheaper and thus available to the poor. Wakley responded that the poor should be told what they were getting for their money.) Another distinguished Victorian writer, Charles Dickens, was moved to take up the cause. He referred many times in his novels and other writings to poor quality food and to fraud, but his most significant action was as editor (1850-59) of the weekly magazine *Household Words*, which ran no less than nine articles dealing with or mentioning food adulteration [4.16].

While prepared to generate comparable publicity in Birmingham by obtaining samples himself, analysing and reporting on them, Postgate also decided on a campaign of direct political lobbying for new legislation. It was fortunate for him that the Birmingham of those days was a political town: its citizens were disposed to take a lively interest in local and national affairs. Meetings on current issues, national or parochial, were well-attended; resolutions would be passed, petitions to Parliament would readily find signatories. The trend was always in a radical direction: favourable towards liberty, free trade, electoral reform, social reforms in general, and the righting of injustices. Debate was lively; in 1840 a 3-day public discussion of socialism, as promulgated by Robert Owen, had drawn nightly audiences of 3000 and led to a bitter argument in the local press about which side had carried the majority. The principles underlying the Chartists' efforts towards universal suffrage had found widespread support in Birmingham during the 1840s, though the often inflammatory speeches and actions of the Chartists themselves were apt to turn moderates towards less radical Reform Bills. When in 1846 the Corn Laws, which had so inflated food prices, were repealed, the event was "celebrated by several public dinners" in Birmingham, at which "the health of Messrs Cobden, Bright and Villiers was drank with much enthusiasm". But Birmingham was by no means parochial; the democratic revolt in Hungary, against the autocracy of the Emperor Ferdinand, initiated in 1848 by Lajos Kossuth, seems especially to have captured the civic imagination: messages of support were sent from Town Meetings and when, in 1851, Kossuth was prevailed upon to visit the town as an official guest, a procession of 60,000 to 70,000 men bearing flags, bunting, trade symbols, augmented with six bands, turned out to welcome him, and the streets were lined with gazers, mostly displaying the Hungarian tricolour. He left with a gift of £750 for his cause [4.17].

Birmingham was clearly receptive soil for reformist causes when Postgate initiated his own campaign. On 7 January, 1854, he wrote a public letter to one of the Members of Parliament for Birmingham, Mr William Scholefield, giving an account of the evils of adulteration and outlining a legislative remedy based on the creation of a Public Analyst. Scholefield (1809-1867) was a highly respected citizen of Birmingham, coming from a political family; he had been Mayor and High Bailiff of the town before gaining his seat in Parliament in 1847 [4.18]. He was a man of high principles; as Mayor he had refused to accept the Town Council's vote of £200 for unexpectedly high expenses during his term of office. Scholefield received Postgate's letter favourably and replied on 9 January:

> "....The evil of adulteration in articles of food is great, and, I am afraid, a growing one, and anyone who can point to an adequate remedy for it will confer an important benefit on the community, and especially on the poorer classes. I am glad, therefore, to see that the subject occupies your attention and shall be pleased if I can so co-operate with you as to lead to a practical check to the frauds now so common. Your suggestion of a public analyser, whose duties, under the conditions you name, shall be analogous to those of the inspectors of weights and measures, inspectors of meat &c., appears to me the best I have seen...." [4.19]

At the same time Postgate had spoken in similar vein to the Mayor of

Birmingham and some members of the Town Council, proposing that the Council establish a Public Analyst to examine foodstuffs through its Borough Improvement Bill. Those he spoke to approved of his remedy in principle, but in the event the Council took no action [4.20].

However, his exchange with Scholefield was encouraging, and in a second letter on 23 January Postgate enlarged upon his ideas:

> "... Perhaps I had better state the plan in more detail. 1.-The appointment of a Public Analyst should rest with the Town Council. His duties to be to purchase, or cause to be purchased without notice, at any shop, articles of food, groceries, drugs &c., for examination and analysis. and report in case of adulteration to the magistrates, who shall have – secondly, a discretionary power of inflicting a fine after hearing the evidence of the public analyser. No legal definition or act of parliament could secure an article from adulteration for long, for as soon as a substance was found to be mixed with an article and declared to be adulterated and illegal, another would be substituted for it, so great and prolific is the ingenuity of fraud in these matters. The decision of adulteration, however defined, must rest with the public analyser..." [4.19]

The letter went on to explain that, though his plan gave rather a lot of power to the Public Analyst, he would be an appointee of the Town Council and subject to enquiry in the event of a wrong decision.

Again Scholefield concurred, and Postgate set about rallying additional parliamentary support for his plan. He enlisted Mr Spooner, the MP for North Warwickshire, by purchasing samples of food and drugs locally and demonstrating the presence of adulterants. Spooner agreed to support Scholefield in parliament. He also wrote to Mr George Muntz, the outspoken second Member for Birmingham, who discussed the matter with Scholefield but remained doubtful about the practical workings of any such plan; responding on 1 February 1854 to a letter from Postgate, Muntz wrote:

> ".... I am at present at a loss to see how any law will prevent [the evil] without being an interference with trade which would not be submitted to. I will, however, assist my colleague as far as I reasonably can...."

Postgate's reply stressed the points that only dishonest traders would have anything to fear, and that a public analyst would be a positive protection to honest traders, who could call upon him if they were doubtful about something received from a wholesaler. He added that "several men in business", who resented competition from traders who sold adulterated articles, viewed his proposal in that light.

Scholefield considered that some press publicity would be advantageous, as a means of mobilising sufficient public feeling to command parliament's attention. Accordingly, for April of that year, Postgate organised a conference on adulteration for the scientific and medical community of Birmingham at which his proposals for legislation would be presented and discussed. The nature and objectives of the meeting were announced approvingly in *The Birmingham Mercury*, *The Midland Counties Herald*, *Aris's Birmingham Gazette* and in *The Times* and other London papers. Scholefield took the Chair. The meeting was a success; the topic of food and drugs adulteration was well aired and the conference passed a number of resolutions stemming from Postgate's proposals. These need not be recorded *in extenso* here; in essence they set out the evils of adulteration; pointed out that science could now detect such fraud; endorsed Postgate's proposal for fines by magistrates based on reports of "public Analysers" – but cases involving wholesalers to be referred to County courts; requested the M.P.s for Birmingham (Scholefield and Muntz) to bring the matter before the House of Commons; and finally expressed thanks to the press for its support, to John Postgate for his zeal and legislative proposals, and to the Editor of *The Lancet* for "his able exposure of this monstrous abuse". *The Lancet* published an account of the meeting.

What should be the next step? Despite his teaching commitments, and the demands of his practice, and undistracted by the birth of his first son, John Percival, in 1853 and a short-lived daughter, Mary Ann, two years later, Postgate started canvassing support. He wrote to cabinet ministers, M.P.s, civic authorities, scientists and others; he promulgated meetings in other towns and cities, sometimes visiting them himself so that, having arranged for samples to be purchased locally, he could demonstrate the presence of adulterants. He found a particularly positive response in Wolverhampton, where a committee in aid of his campaign was formed, with Alfred Hall Browne as its Hon. Secretary. He and Browne concocted a circular letter to the whole of the medical profession, and enlisted *The Lancet*'s help in publicising it [4.21]. The letter informed his fellow professionals that Scholefield would take up the matter of adulteration in parliament, asked them to consider forming town committees to petition the House in favour of legislation, and offered appropriate advice and information. It was accompanied by a summary of the evils of adulteration and the injuries thereby inflicted, the concluding paragraph of which read:

> "...the whole subject demands the serious consideration of the community, as a question deeply concerning public health, and urgently requires the interference of the Legislature to suppress practices which involve gross impositions on society, and especially on the poorer classes."

But more direct political action was also needed. Scholefield was willing to introduce a Bill in the House of Commons forthwith, but Postgate took the view that this was premature. He favoured the setting up, by the House, of a Select Committee to enquire into the whole field of adulteration – covering food, drink and drugs; and to take expert evidence which would make the scandalous situation absolutely clear to all: M.P.s, the legislature, the medical profession and the public. However, it was Scholefield who had to take the necessary action, and initially his view prevailed. Tactfully, Postgate concurred, only sending Scholefield a detailed letter outlining the problems that the Bill would have to take into account. Who should pay the Public Analysts? What should be done about recidivist fraudulent traders? Who should be held responsible for fraud originating with a wholesaler? Was compensation a public issue, if so, payable to whom and by whom? What should be done about fraudulent mis-prescription of drugs? (The latter item arose from the experience of a medical friend, in which the druggist had systematically omitted the crucial ingredient of a prescription for one of the doctor's patients. There was at the time no legal remedy for such fraud at all.) The letter had the effect Postgate had probably foreseen: Scholefield, doubtless impressed by the need to have irrefutable data as a basis for effective legislation, changed his stance with but little further argument. He abandoned his plan for a Bill and agreed instead to move for a Select Committee of Enquiry in the House. He did so on 26 June, 1855.

The food reformists were by now very unpopular with the more conservative elements of society, especially among the "evil-hearted grocers" (G K Chesterton), and it was probably fortunate that, largely because of anxieties over the conduct of the Crimean War, the conservative coalition administration headed by Lord Aberdeen had just been replaced on 5 February of that year by a Liberal majority led by Lord Palmerston. Parliament agreed, and forthwith appointed a Committee of fifteen M.P.s, including Scholefield as chairman, to conduct the enquiry.

Chapter 5

THE SELECT COMMITTEE

The Select Committee of Enquiry into the Adulterations of Food, Drink and Drugs got down to business on 13 July, 1855, and very business-like it was. The minutes show that it held eight meetings between then and 8 August, taking evidence from seventeen witnesses. It produced two provisional reports and assembled again on more than a dozen occasions between February and May, 1856, [5.1] interviewing another forty witnesses, producing thereafter its final report. Some witnesses were called more than once; Postgate was called on three occasions. Appropriately, the first witness of all was Hassall, whose evidence amounted to a wide-ranging and detailed survey of his work for *The Lancet*. It occupied a lot of the Committee's time that day, included a brief explanation of his microscopical techniques, and must have been devastating for any Committee member who was not already aware of the scale of adulteration in mid-century Britain. Equally appropriately, as the senior and most productive exposer of adulteration, Hassall was recalled to be the last witness as well.

Witnesses were drawn from many walks of life. They included Professors of Chemistry, Pharmacy and Medical Jurisprudence; a lawyer; physicians and surgeons; officials of the Board of Inland Revenue, of the Post Office, and of the Mustard Department of Her Majesty's Victualling Yard; Board of Health officers from London and near Manchester; the Mayor of Dublin; several druggists (wholesale and retail); a food manufacturer; numerous professional analysts; a licencer of apothecaries; authorities on brewing and drug manufacture; three journal editors; a grocer; tea brokers; three bakers; a miller...

Among the editors, Wakley was naturally called; he was among the 1856 witnesses and, since Hassall had presented the *The Lancet*'s Commission's findings in detail, Wakley's evidence was brief, largely emphasising the scale of adulterative fraud and the need for controls. The editor of the *Pharmaceutical Journal* gave evidence that adulteration of drugs was widely practised (this problem had been reported to parliament as early as 1834 by Richard Phillips FRS, who also gave evidence); and the editor of the *Reformer's Gazette*, a Glasgow paper, told of threats made to him when he publicised a case of adulteration of oatmeal with bran and husks.

A revealing interview was that with Thomas Blackwell, of Crosse and Blackwell, the pickle and preserve manufacturers (still extant in 1996). He described candidly how his firm had until recently manufactured green pickles. Pickled vegetables are not naturally green, so the firm's practice had been to boil

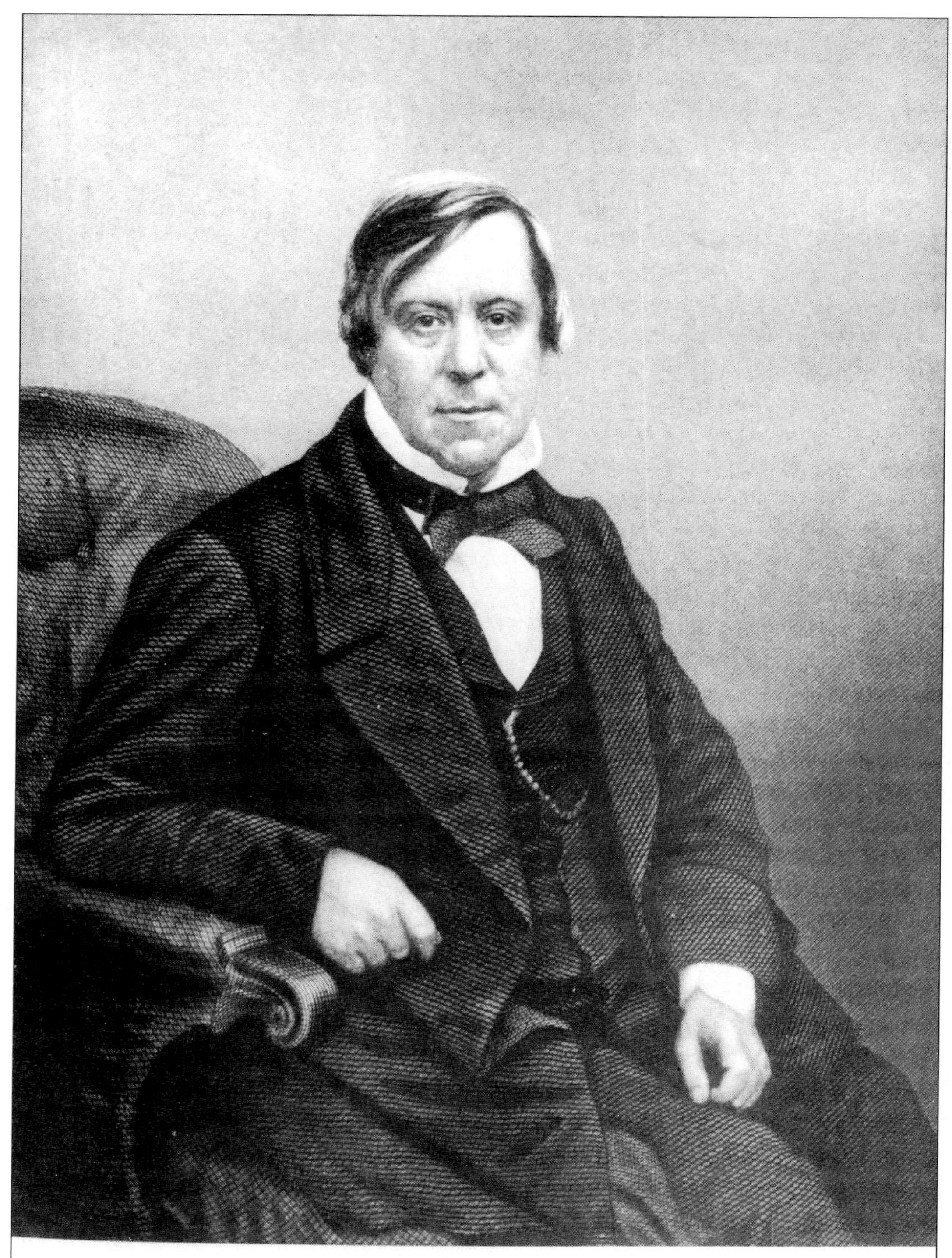

William Scholefield, Charter Mayor, 1838; M.P. 1847–67

the vinegar (which is essentially dilute acetic acid) in copper vats three times, when it became green because some of the copper dissolved as copper acetate. This is a green substance which was even then known to be poisonous. The liquor so formed imparted a green colour to the vegetables pickled in it by staining them with copper acetate. When The Lancet exposed the dangers inherent in consuming such pickles, the firm behaved, in Hassall's words, "in a most honourable manner", and discontinued the practice, using glass-lined vessels instead. They lost a lot of customers, and, to Blackwell's expressed astonishment, received many letters of complaint from the public. The affair of the green pickles, and gooseberries dyed green, as reported amusingly in *The Times*, ("Green as it was, however, it seems that the consumers were still greener...") dismayed Charles Dickens [5.2], though he seems not to have grasped that both the Committee and Mr Blackwell were opposed to such practices.

The fact that the public often demanded food and drinks with colours, consistencies or prices which could not be sustained without additives, ie: adulterants, illustrates one of the Committee's problems. Another was the matter (mentioned earlier) of adding chicory to coffee, which led to a cheaper and hence more widely available beverage. Addition of chicory was in fact legal, and a witness, Charles Burton, described how he had seen chicory powdered and compressed into "berries" having the same shape and colour as coffee "berries" (today known as "coffee beans"). The Committee concurred with Wakley's earlier comment in Parliament: chicory would be an acceptable additive provided its presence was made clear, quantitatively, to the customer.

Another witness, a lawyer, pressed the point that there were a number of "adulterants" which improved the appearance or keeping qualities of foodstuffs or drugs, and argued that there was no need to inform the public of their presence provided they were harmless; on the contrary, to do so interfered with what we should today call market forces. If the public liked such a product, it was to the competitive advantage of the trader that he provide it. Professor of Chemistry Theophilus Redwood was somewhat critical of Hassall's findings, though he did not deny the evils or the prevalence of deliberate adulteration; he had earlier advised the Committee to distinguish between conventional adulterants, such as hops in beer, and fraudulent ones, and had also made the point that many ingredients used in food, drinks and drugs were not pure substances in the chemical sense; surely such materials could legitimately be used if experience had shown that their impurities were harmless?

The evidence of Mr Alphonse Normandy indicated a new difficulty for the Committee. He had spoken to the Committee on the adulteration of drugs, giving some details of samples of sodium bicarbonate most of which proved to be contaminated with sodium sulphate. After his evidence had been made public he had sought new samples, and all of them proved to be pure. He had also sought to purchase samples of chocolate for checking from a "large seller", who had refused to supply him. Apparently the Committee's publicity was causing a reaction among at least some traders, who were concealing dubious wares from members, or providing specially pure samples. Yet Mr Thomas Herring, a druggist witness, strongly favoured inspection and regulation of drugs. Indeed, though the druggists and pharmacists were inclined to play down the incidence of drug adulteration, and tended to blame 'drug grinders' rather than vendors for such cases as existed, they were generally in favour of regulation in principle. Not so one of the grocers, Mr James Abbiss, who asserted that adulteration of tea was rare and readily detectable by the public, and that coffee adulterated with chicory was better, price for price, than pure coffee. Two tea brokers also maintained that adulteration of tea was by then rare, contradicting the evidence of analyst witnesses.

Bread and flour provoked controversy. Many witnesses told of the widespread use of alum (sodium aluminium sulphate) in bread (a matter amplified in John Postgate's evidence below), but one of the bakers maintained doggedly that, in London, such adulteration was rare and under control. In contrast, two witnesses were managers of co-operative enterprises (in Rochdale and Leeds) which had come together to supply their members with unadulterated bread, so little did they trust their local bakers; the one in Leeds supplied 33,000 people.

Another baker's evidence was sad, and shows *The Lancet*'s Analytical Commission in a poor light. He was indignant because he had been named in *The Lancet* for selling bread adulterated with alum; consequently he had lost business and, convinced that he was innocent, had tried to get his sample back from Wakley for independent analysis. Wakley had high-handedly refused. One hopes it was a rare case.

An important witness was Dr Henry Letheby, who was called on 8 August (immediately after Postgate's second interview, below). Letheby was an analytical chemist then working at the London Hospital who had, a few years earlier, been employed by Wakley and Hassall's Commission for some confirmatory analyses of tobacco, snuff and opium. Like several other witnesses, he distinguished between accidental and fraudulent adulteration, taking the reasonable view that much accidental adulteration was inescapable and generally harmless. In his experience, the adulteration of confectionery was the most dangerous of the fraudulent practices then current. He told of a street vendor who, in 1853, had bought rejects from a reputable confectioner's establishment and then sold them in Petticoat Lane. They poisoned 24 people:

they proved to have been dyed yellow with toxic lead chromate (happily all the cases recovered, but they were in real danger).

John Postgate's first interview took place on 1 August, 1855, [5.3] fairly early in the Committee's programme. It was concerned wholly with the adulteration of flour and the sale of adulterated bread. Among common adulterants were bean flour, starch, potato flour and alum. Bean and potato flour, and presumably starch, were simply cheaper than wheat flour and their covert use was simply cheating; alum was used as a whitener and was more dangerous. Postgate had had in his house bread containing 3.5% alum, but that was exceptional. More commonly it would contain some 0.25% alum; he had eaten such bread and he described its toxicity:

> "The gums become swollen; the tongue more or less so. There is an unpleasant taste in the mouth, and the stomach itself becomes affected. There is a quantity of acid secreted and the individual suffers from an attack of dyspepsia...."

He added the opinion that its toxic effects were cumulative. He, too, pointed to the paradox caused by uneducated public taste: that when a bakery in Birmingham set out to supply a wholesome alum-free bread, its customers complained that the bread was yellowish in colour; "they [the bakers] had considerable difficulty in establishing their business."

The Chairman reminded him that adulteration of flour was in fact illegal under an existing Act of Parliament, with substantial fines as penalties; Postgate quickly pointed out, "But you have no person to detect those adulterations." He went on to indicate briefly the need for official Public Analysts, but time was running out and he was unable to outline his ideas in detail – indeed, it was probably inappropriate at this stage of the Committee's deliberations as it had many witnesses yet to interview. The Committee generated a touch of light relief in their concluding questions, which concerned the punishment appropriate to a fraudulent baker. Postgate was asked:

> "Would you adopt the French system of suspending tradesmen for a time?" – "I think a distinction should be drawn between pernicious and harmless adulteration; harmless adulteration I should consider a swindle; but I think a person guilty of pernicious adulteration ought to be imprisoned."
> "With a little hard labour, perhaps?" – "Yes, and the more educated the criminal, the greater should be the punishment. The practice of adulteration is a practice for the benefit of the party resorting to it at the expense of the purchaser."
> "Would it not be desirable to make him eat his own bread in his imprisonment?" – "Yes, and leave him to reflect on its effects."

At his second interview on 3 August, although he mentioned having received fresh samples of adulterated bread (from Wolverhampton), he was able to talk about a wider range of adulterations. Adulterated mustard, a matter later discussed in detail by the official from Her Majesty's Victualling Yard, was not just a gastronomic problem: mustard poultices were widely used in medicine, and if the mustard contained turmeric, the most common additive, they were less effective. He also spoke of red lead (a slow but cumulative poison) being found in cayenne pepper, but on the whole he concerned himself with impure and adulterated drugs: quinine diluted with salicin, cod liver oil diluted with bland oils, castor oil containing a very violent purgative, potassium iodide (used for iodine tinctures) contaminated with potassium carbonate. All these caused dosages to be mis-prescribed and could endanger patients' lives or delay their recovery. He quoted a letter he had received from the Principal of Sydenham College, a practising physician at Birmingham General Hospital, who, after congratulating him on his efforts before the Committee, stated:

> "[From] my experience in the treatment of acute diseases ... I believe many lives have been lost when adulterated drugs have been relied upon."

On his third appearance before the Committee, after being asked to report (briefly, the Chairman emphasised) on new examples of adulteration that he had come across, which he did, he was invited to explain at length his ideas on the sort of legislation which he thought was now needed.

First he proposed that an Order in Council should be issued at once prohibiting injurious, pernicious and fraudulent adulteration, the vendors being held responsible, pending a special Act of Parliament. The Act should include the following features.

1. From time to time a central body, such as the Board of Health, should provide guidelines and definitions of what constituted adulterants.
2. That a network of Public Analysts should be set up. (He offered views on what the titles and qualifications of such Officers should be).
3. That the Officer should be appointed and financed by the local authority but be independent in his activities, and his salary be independent of these, too.
4. That he should purchase, or cause to be purchased, samples of articles to be analysed, and undertake their analysis. These could include linen, cloth and silk, as well as food, drinks and drugs. He should also analyse substances at the request of traders, for a fee to be payable to the local authority. That authority should hold securely for a time a portion of any sample analysed, in case of dispute.

5. Penalties should be imposed by magistrates and the Officer should give evidence when required.
6. He should be empowered to make inspections of shops and stores whose owners had been subject to previous convictions.
7. There should be registers of traders, with lists published half-yearly. Habitual offenders would be refused registration and their names published.

He amplified several of these points during his presentation and explained their purposes and merits. The Committee then cross-examined him in detail about how his plans would work in practice: how many public analysts would be needed to bring adulteration under control? How much would they and their analytical procedures cost? What could be done about imports which were adulterated overseas? How should standards of purity and/or freedom from additives be decided upon and promulgated? These and many other questions he fielded easily, for he had clearly thought the matter through in great detail; only on the financial side was he vague. A big town such as Birmingham would manage with one analyst, who would cost some £500 per annum; this could be met, he thought, out of fines and fees.

The enquiry had been exhaustive, and doubtless exhausting for the Committee members, because the same ground often had to be gone over again and again with different witnesses. The Committee accepted (as did Hassall and Postgate) that two varieties of adulteration could be distinguished, deleterious adulteration, which was not only fraudulent but also damaging to the health or well-being of the consumer, and innocuous adulteration, which, being harmless, could sometimes make for a cheaper product and at worst was simply fraud. (This distinction aroused the wrath of *The Times* which, though generally supportive of the Committee's ideas, felt that to treat innocuous adulteration softly was to open the door to "pernicious adulteration". In either case the public was at the mercy of the shopkeepers.) The upshot was a quite appalling catalogue of evidence to the effect that, though adulteration had diminished significantly since *The Lancet* had publicised its findings so dramatically, it was still rife throughout the country – indeed accepted as a fact of life by many people. The lawyer and a minority of the traders were the only witnesses to question the need for firmer regulation; the rest were in favour, many of them vehemently so.

The Committee appeared to be wholly in sympathy with Postgate's proposed remedies. It produced its final report after the end of its last sittings on 22 July, 1856, and his ideas formed the gist of its recommendations.

Chapter 6

ITS AFTERMATH

The evidence presented to Scholefield's Committee of Enquiry "was widely circulated throughout the Empire, and it created a great impression on the public mind." [6.1]. For example, the issue of Charles Dickens's *Household Words* for March 22, 1856, carried a long article on 'Poison' by Henry Morley, its general message being that science was providing new and effective ways of detecting poisons. It alluded to the adulteration of food and drugs in terms which might almost have been a digest of Postgate's views:

> "To sell an article for what it is not is a fraud – a lie; and it is indisputable that the suppression of all secret and intentional adulteration would be not merely a great gain to society, but a great gain to the interests of trade. To detect and punish such adulteration is as much a duty to just-minded tradesmen as to those who buy of them; and to suppress at least poisonous adulteration, if it be possible to be done, is a distinct obligation on the state, of which to protect life is by no means the least important function. A permanent committee of five or six persons, who possess the best attainable knowledge of chemistry, botany and natural history, aided by a simple machinery of detection, and subordinated, perhaps to the General Board of Health, might not only keep down all practices of deleterious adulteration, but might even supply particular trades with a great many of those points of scientific information which they have not yet turned to the right account."[6.2]

At the parliamentary level the next step was clearly to build upon the Committee's report, hoping to strike while its impact was still fresh. Postgate briefed Scholefield to enable him to introduce a bill, one which would not cover all the issues raised, but would make the adulteration of food a crime punishable by six months' imprisonment, and would establish a staff of officers to carry out the Act's provisions. Drug adulteration, for instance, would not be brought into this Act at all. However, so great were the pressures on Parliament's time that even this relatively unambitious bill was not read until 25 June, 1857. It encountered immense opposition. Food traders massed in protest in the lobby of the House of Commons, and such was their influence on individual members that not a single M.P. spoke in defence of the bill. Scholefield was greatly disheartened; the bill had to be withdrawn without achieving a second reading. Meanwhile a new consequence of the situation in Britain had become apparent:

the adulterated state of drugs and other articles imported from Britain had become so bad that in 1856 the Spanish Cortes had been moved to pass its own adulteration act [6.3].

John Postgate was nothing if not stubborn. Despite the disappointment over Scholefield's bill he announced that, "as long as he could get a member to move in the House of Commons, or a newspaper to publish his addresses and testings, he would continue the work until Parliament provided an efficient law." [6.4]. While the Commission of Enquiry had been taking evidence he had kept the topic in the public eye, with circulars and letters to the press. He participated in meetings all over the North of England – for example, at Lincoln, Scarborough, Wakefield, Leeds, Bradford, Dudley, Wolverhampton – usually by invitation of the Mayor or citizens in the professions, and he assisted with their organisation. Samples of locally purchased foods, shown to be adulterated, would be displayed. As a trained analyst he did many of the analyses himself; he had told Scholefield's Committee of Enquiry that, "To make a rough estimate, perhaps two thirds of the articles have been found to be adulterated in the towns that I have visited." On 29 February 1856, after the Committee of Enquiry's second interim report, he had called together and addressed, at the request of the Mayor of Birmingham, a meeting in the Town hall to discuss the evidence presented to the Committee so far. After a discussion in which two resolutions were passed, one expressing alarm at the prevalence of adulteration, the other calling for counter-measures, the meeting unanimously adopted the following petition to the House of Commons, to be presented by their M.P., Mr Scholefield; copies were sent to the Prime Minister and Home Secretary:

The humble petition of the inhabitants of Birmingham,
in town's meeting assembled,

> *Sheweth,* – That your petitioners are assured that the adulteration of articles of food and medicine is carried on to an alarming extent throughout the kingdom of Great Britain and Ireland. That such a system seriously affects the health and physical condition of Her Majesty's subjects generally, and that the means hitherto employed have failed to repress the evil. That it is of the greatest importance to the moral well-being of the trading classes of this community that a system so subversive of the first principles of honesty, and so seriously involving the character of the people, should, if possible, be put an end to. That your petitioners humbly implore your House to take the subject into your serious consideration, and to provide some remedy whereby the evils complained of may be effectually removed. And your petitioners will ever pray, &c."

Postgate continued his own campaign. In 1857 he published a polemical pamphlet entitled *'A Few Words on Adulteration'* [6.5], giving examples of the toxic effects of adulterants drawn from all over the country, pointing out the action of the Spanish Cortes mentioned earlier, and writing angrily of the need to legislate against the "nefarious dealer who, utterly regardless of everything except his fraudulent gains and his own safety in obtaining them, scruples not to introduce the most potent poisons into articles of food whenever it suits his purpose to do so".

In that year he also helped to arrange a national meeting in Birmingham. It was the inaugural meeting of the National Association for the Promotion of Social Science. This was a 3-day meeting (13-15 October) at which Lord Brougham, its President, gave the opening address, and it had sections dealing with Jurisprudence, Education, Punishment and Reform, and Public Health. Among numerous invited papers presented on many aspects of public affairs, sixteen were by Birmingham authors. A *soirée* and *conversazione* were also held. Postgate read a paper to the Public Health section, predictably on "The Adulteration of Food and Drugs", which included the proposals he had made to the Scholefield Committee. It was later published in the Association's Transactions [6.6]. He was "highly complimented" on his contribution by the President of his section, Lord Stanley, and by Lord Brougham, who agreed with his proposals for legislation and encouraged him to take further action despite the opposition he had so far encountered. That opposition had extended even to the present meeting: according to a biographical sketch of his life published many years later [6.7], "an effort was made to prevent [Postgate's paper] being read". How, by whom and why were not stated, but presumably food and drug traders were behind the effort.

The published version of his paper was, for its period, remarkably brisk and to the point, at least at its outset, for he was covering utterly familiar ground. In a series of short paragraphs he indicated, with real examples, six reasons why adulteration of comestibles and drugs was practised. They were: to make spurious substitutes; to increase bulk or weight; to restore deteriorated appearance; to improve a naturally poor appearance; to dye; to add flavour. He followed these with a catalogue of examples of such adulteration, drawn partly from the evidence heard by Scholefield's Committee of Enquiry, partly from his own investigations, and emphasised that it was at its worst in country villages and poor neighbourhoods. He then discussed, again with examples, the social consequences of adulteration in terms of public morals, public health, revenue and commerce. Finally he discussed remedies, outlining his concept of a network of public analysts. His passage on the impact of widespread adulteration on public morals displays his outlook well, for all its convoluted expression;

> "When the trading classes are engaged as a body in the practice of adulteration, juveniles may be reformed and criminals locked up, nevertheless a large portion of society is cankered to the core. All the precepts and principles instilled by benevolence into the former are slowly removed, and callousness to rectitude of conduct induced; and, as regards the locked-up criminal, by what right of justice is he to be confined whilst the aggregate crimes of intelligent capitalists go unpunished."

A timeless message that applies far beyond adulteration!

By 1859 Postgate had persuaded Scholefield to resume the fight. Their new strategy was to get a deliberately weak bill passed which would be the thin end of a wedge, so to speak, since it could be amended and toughened later. Postgate actually drew up the text of this bill (as, it seems, he did with later ones [6.8]); all it did was empower local authorities, in England only, to appoint Public Analysts; it set limits to the modest charges they would make for analyses on behalf of the public, and prescribed modest penalties for sellers of adulterated goods. To bring adulteration before the public again, as a precursor to the presentation of the bill, Postgate arranged with the Mayor of Birmingham to call another town meeting, a large one, on 28 January. At this he again spoke on adulteration in general, and tested and displayed adulterants in many articles purchased in the town. A resolution was passed calling for Postgate's proposals as adopted by Scholefield's Committee – a network of municipal public analysts and stringent penalties – to become law.

However, it was the new bill Scholefield introduced on 29 February. It was so mild that it got through to the committee stage where, on 25 July, it was amended. Presumably the parliamentary session then ran out of time; there was a delay of several months. It was re-introduced in an amended form, causing it to apply to the whole of Great Britain, in April of 1860. Despite its weak character, it would probably have been rejected but for a particularly gruesome case of adulteration which came to light in Bradford. A druggist's assistant was instructed to adulterate peppermint lozenges with plaster of Paris (calcium sulphate – a fairly harmless fraud) and used white arsenic (arsenic trioxide – a powerful poison) instead. More than thirty people are said to have died as a result. On a wave of public revulsion the bill was passed, and received Royal Assent in July, as the Adulteration Act of 1860 (more correctly, the Act of Parliament for the Prevention of the Adulteration of Food or Drink by Local Authorities 1860).

It was a weak act in the sense that it was left to each municipality to decide whether or not it wanted a public analyst, and most were unlikely to do anything about it at all. Postgate had tried to get its penalties strengthened when it passed

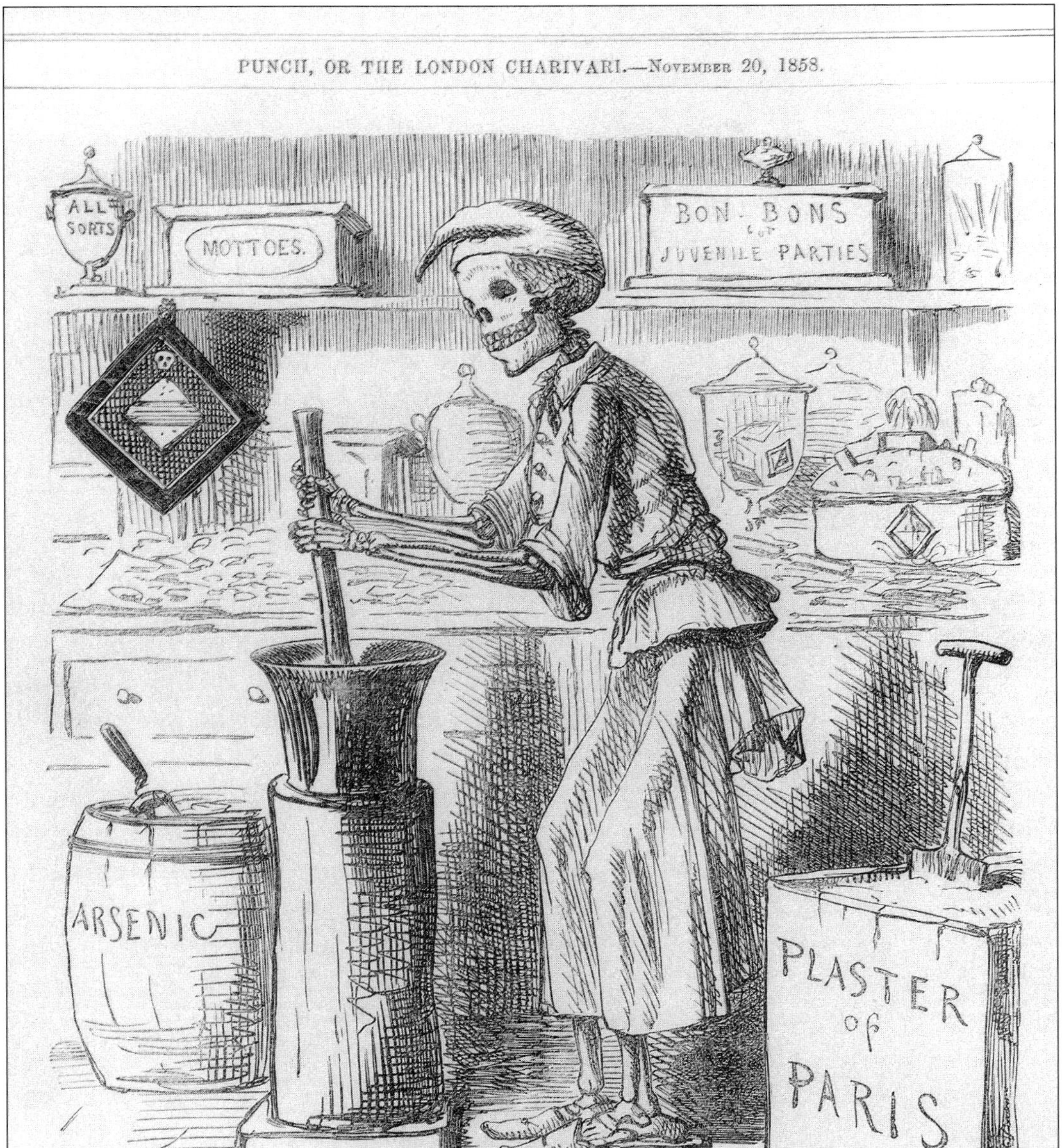

PUNCH, OR THE LONDON CHARIVARI.—November 20, 1858.

THE GREAT LOZENGE-MAKER.

A Hint to Paterfamilias.

Punch*'s main cartoon for a week in November, 1858, p207.*

through the House of Lords; he provided the Earl of Shaftesbury with two draft clauses to this effect. But the plan was abandoned: for the Lords to return it to the Commons with a radical amendment was politically too risky, as it might have led to the whole bill being rejected.

Within weeks of the 1860 Act coming into force, and after consulting him informally, Postgate wrote an open letter to the Mayor of Birmingham, Thomas Lloyd, drawing his attention to the Act and urging his Council to put it into operation. The letter was reported verbatim in the *British Medical Journal* [6.9], and is a little curious in that a substantial part is devoted to outlining the history of the Act and his own part in it, and pointing out, quite correctly, that the provisions of the Act and the political agitation for it originated in Birmingham.

> "I mention these matters, because I have observed a disposition to filch credit from Birmingham by taking it from the originator and workers of this question", he wrote cryptically.

That the letter was published in the *British Medical Journal* and not in *The Lancet* might be significant. Could Wakley and Hassall have come to resent the energy and political success of the younger agitator? Or can others have belittled Scholefield's and Postgate's political efforts? This paragraph is an early hint that credit was not always being given where it was due in this affair.

In Birmingham yet another town meeting was called, presided over by the Mayor, then Alderman Manton, and a resolution was passed urging the Corporation to appoint an analyst. In due course this was done, and Birmingham at last had its official Public Analyst. Support for the official was not unanimous; many traders were incensed and, in the words of J A Langford, historian of Birmingham, "attempts were made to abolish the office of analyst in Birmingham annually – fortunately without result..." [6.10]. Analysts were also appointed in some other towns, including Dublin, Sheffield, the City of London and some of the Metropolitan districts. By the winter of 1860, Postgate's political activities were beginning to show results.

In 1860 the academic side of his career took a step upward: on 7 May he was appointed Professor of Medical Jurisprudence and Toxicology in Queens College, lecturing in both the legal and medical departments. And at home his family had grown. A second daughter, Isabella Jane, had arrived in 1856, and a third, Agnes Foord, in 1857 – but in that year the young Mary Ann had died. A second son, John, was born in 1859; the doctor's wife had much to occupy her. By 1861 the family had moved house from Belmont Row to the Edgbaston district, further from the centre of Birmingham.

The Act of 1860 was not only weak. It seems that some authorities found it, or regarded it as, difficult to work. Postgate did what he could to clarify its provisions and explain how it was intended to work. He sent a public letter to the authorities, the gist of which was printed in the *British Medical Journal* in August, 1861 [6.11]. It is worth quoting in some detail because, allowing for Victorian punctuation, it reveals his personal determination to make the best of the Act, his concern for the poor, the precision of his thought on legal matters, and also his by now proprietary feeling about the campaign for legislation. After asserting the importance of the Act both to the public and to tradespeople, he wrote:

> "... Persistently agitating the question until the measure was obtained, and part of my suggestions forming, in fact, its base, I beg to offer a few remarks on the subject.
>
> "No doubt the Act is not all I desired or asked for; still under it – fairly, honestly and energetically worked – the public have an efficient remedy for the enormous evil of adulteration; and the fair, honourable, and legitimate trader may free himself from the dishonest competition of his fraudulent neighbour, and have a sure means (at a small cost) of knowing the nature of the commodities he purchases for retail...
>
> "The power which this Act gives to local bodies to appoint public analysers to whom all purchasers, the public and traders alike, may apply, is a great step .. [which] .. even without proceedings before the magistrate, must tend directly to diminish adulteration.
>
> "Much misconception prevails, I find, respecting the first clause of the Act. That clause makes two offences – one, that of selling, knowingly, commodities adulterated with substances injurious to health, and would, of course, require proof of such knowledge before conviction.; but the other strikes at the root of the mischief, and places a remedy in the hands of the public; for it expressly states, "Every person who shall sell as pure or unadulterated any article of food or drink, which is adulterated or not pure, shall for every such offence forfeit and pay a penalty not exceeding £5, with costs; and, for a second offence, the name and residence of the offender may be advertised, at his expense, in the newspapers." It is therefore perfectly clear, ... that purchasers have only to ask for the pure article, and request the seller to label it as such; and equally is it clear that impure and adulterated articles of food or drink must be sold as such; but even these may bring the seller under the law, should they contain any material harmful to health...[the magistrates would not have admitted a plea of ignorance, the services of the public analyser being now available to all – author].
>
> ".... the suppression of adulteration now rests with the local authorities.

> The efficiency or non-efficiency of the Act depends entirely on the amount of public spirit possessed by corporations. If .. [they] .. are determined to enforce the measure and carry it out vigorously, they can do so by ordering inspectors of meat and markets to procure and submit samples of articles of food to the analyser for examination, and initiate the proceedings before the magistrates..."

The letter went on to point out that if, as in Birmingham, the analyst were paid by salary, and not by fees, the corporation could, for the public good, choose to remit fees, or give the analyst discretionary power to investigate cases without charge himself.

> "Corporate action is much needed in this matter to protect the poor artisan, who can afford neither the half-crown nor the time wherewith to protect himself. It is, therefore, to be hoped that it will be guided by broad principles of public duty...
> "As regards the retail dealer, he is, doubtless, generally speaking, quite competent to take care of himself. The Act abundantly protects him. [He could now use the analyst's services, cheaply – author.] He should order pure articles; have them invoiced as such; and aid the authorities to suppress adulteration, by proceeding against parties who have sold him sophisticated food."

Even as he wrote, Postgate clearly saw the weaknesses of the Act as it stood: local authorities had no obligation to take any action at all. Since traders were often influential members of local government Councils or Corporations, a great many authorities would choose to do nothing. He continued to lecture about adulteration and the new Act; the *British Medical Journal* reported at some length a typical lecture given in Bridlington late in 1861 [6.12]. But it was clear to him that he must take further political steps to make implementation of the Act compulsory. In addition, a glaring gap existed which needed plugging: drug adulteration should be brought under the Act's umbrella.

He approached Scholefield, who agreed to introduce a bill which would amend the Act accordingly. Bringing in drugs would be the easier matter, so Postgate drafted an appropriate bill and sent it to Scholefield on 10 September 1863. Scholefield was well satisfied with the draft, and felt strongly in its favour, but his health was deteriorating and he was unable to make progress with it. In effect his poor health put a stop to Postgate's parliamentary lobbying for four years, to his own frustration and also that of Scholefield, who was equally anxious to get on with it. In 1867 one of Birmingham's seats in the House became vacant and John Bright was elected, he of Reform Bill fame, who was in addition a superb Parliamentary speaker. Postgate approached Bright and he proved to be an ally: he undertook to help Scholefield as best he could. In the event, Scholefield died in April of that year, but his successor, George Dixon, agreed to continue his efforts and to present a revised version of the bill. This would have obliged local authorities to appoint analysts; it also covered drugs, and it hardened penalties, prescribing prison sentences for offenders. Dixon introduced it on 9 June, 1868, and it got through to a second reading on 23 June. Then the House of Commons went into recess and the bill lapsed.

Postgate resumed the sort of political agitation with which he had backed up the Act of 1860. He invited M.P.s concerned with the bill to his home and demonstrated the presence of adulterants in locally-purchased food and drugs. He took advantage of another meeting of the National Association for the Promotion of Social Science, the second to be held in Birmingham, to present a paper about the state of legislation on the adulteration of food, drink and drugs [6.13], after which the Association passed a resolution asking its Council to continue its efforts to promote more efficient legislation. George Dixon also raised the matter with the Birmingham Chamber of Commerce, and his speech, with a copy of the bill, was circulated to Chambers of Commerce throughout the country. He re-introduced the bill, somewhat modified, on 13 April 1869, but once again it met with such hostility that he had to withdraw it in July. Dixon's special interest was education and, since progress with adulteration was clearly going to be difficult, he felt it necessary to withdraw from presenting Postgate's bills, though he would continue to add his name in support of them.

From the perspective of the present day, the hostility which John Postgate's bills provoked seems disproportionate. No-one doubted the ubiquity of adulteration, even if some disputed its scale; all accepted that it was blatantly fraudulent, and unfair to honest traders as much as to the public; all agreed that it bore down most heavily on the poor; moreover its dangers were well publicised, born out by regular injurious and sometimes fatal accidents. It seems curious that, in an era when British society was tackling the worst evils of the industrial revolution and reform was in the air, attempts to introduce legislation to right such blatant wrongs should arouse such antagonism. But the reforms which we now look back upon with respect, even though many were unsatisfactory compromises, were only won with great difficulty, and met with strong resistance from vested interests. The First Reform Act of 1832, which enfranchised the wealthier bourgeoisie, had been passed in the teeth of opposition from the aristocracy and the clergy and under threat of violent public demonstrations (the carriages of bishops who had voted against its 1831 version were stoned by an angry 'mob'); only in 1842 did Lord Shaftesbury's Mines Act prohibit women and *children under ten* from working underground in the coal mines. The Factory Acts of 1847 and 1850, which limited the working day in textile factories to 10 hours and added Saturday afternoons to the week-end break, had been resisted by employers for some 20 years – and they left conditions in other industries, and the iniquities of child labour, to be dealt with piecemeal. (Charles Kingsley's *Water Babies* is said to have precipitated the Chimney-Sweeper's Act of 1864, actually an ineffectual piece of legislation). It had taken repeated outbreaks of cholera to force the Government to accept sufficient responsibility for public health to establish the General Board of Health and regional Public Health Boards in 1848. But none of these actions was regarded as adequate by reformers, and in the 1850s to '70s revisions and amendments to the various reforms were constantly being proposed. Some such campaigns were to be successful as, for example, the Second Reform Bill of 1867 (which only succeeded after being defeated in 1860 and again in 1865) and the Public Health Act of 1872. In addition there was turbulence about the Educational Code; the status and accreditation of the medical profession; the effectiveness of the police (the 1850s saw a wave of 'garotting', the Victorian equivalent of mugging, in the streets of the capital). This is not to mention foreign policy, which included the problems arising from the one 'little' war of Queen Victoria's otherwise relatively peaceful reign: the Crimea expedition of 1854-56. And there were thousands of more workaday details of public administration and legislation to be dealt with, including questions which seem astonishing today, such as whether Jews should be allowed seats in Parliament. Parliamentary time was indeed at a premium. Getting permission to introduce a bill was difficult enough; ensuring that it would not be "talked out" was equally hazardous.

As far as opposition to legislation over adulteration is concerned, vested interests undoubtedly played an important part, and clearly the ambiguous position in which middlemen – importers and sellers – might find themselves led to anxiety about the actual legislation. But beneath all that there was a less tangible reason for resistance, a feeling that a British Conservative of the 1980s would have understood well. It was antagonism to government interference in trade; a feeling that market forces would take care of things provided the public was watchful. In foreign policy, 'Free Trade' was the flavour of the mid century. Victorian Britain had become perhaps the least restrictive of the trading nations, with but minimal tariffs and import controls, since most had been abolished by 1860. Free trade had been embraced by Palmerston, Gladstone, Bright and, indeed, all but a minority of both Whig and Tory politicians, and in the 1870s it was being abundantly vindicated, underpinning an economic boom which was the envy of much of Europe. By a sort of spill-over, the idea of interfering with internal trade, of introducing penalties and inspections, was unpalatable. The public ought to take care of itself, and if it did not, it deserved what it got – even if it was toxic, lily-white bread. *Caveat emptor*! Laws already existed to curb the worst excesses of fraud; the public should use them. John Postgate's perfectly sound contention that the poor had not the time, knowledge or spare cash to instigate legal action would have made little impression in that climate. He still had much work to do.

Scholefield had presented five of Postgate's bills, the third of which became the 1860 Act, and Dixon had presented two. (Each time a bill was withdrawn, its re-presentation, always to some extent modified, counted as the presentation of a new bill.) They had done sterling work for the cause. Scholefield had been a willing companion-in-arms, but his health had ultimately let him down; Dixon, one senses, had been a dutiful substitute. But Postgate's third ally proved to be as energetic and as enthusiastic as Postgate himself. Philip Henry Muntz, son of George Muntz (who died in 1857) was M.P. for Warwickshire. He was a subtle and accomplished parliamentarian who understood the many pitfalls of parliamentary procedure – though he could not always avoid them.

J A Langford, in his meticulous record of mid-century life in Birmingham published in 1887 [6.14], gave a blow-by-blow account of Muntz's ultimately successful piloting of an effective Act through parliament. To summarize, once Muntz had agreed to take over from Dixon late in 1869, Postgate had a long talk with him about the problem in general, and left yet another draft of the bill for him to study. Muntz approved of it, and duly brought it before Parliament in February of 1870, where it survived its first reading. It was due for a second reading early in March, when its opponents embarked on parliamentary sabotage. As *The Times* reported next day:

"The second reading of the Adulteration of Food and Drink Act (1860) Amendment Bill was moved by Mr Muntz, but opposed by Mr Bruce, on the ground that there was no time to discuss it. Mr Muntz replied that the bill had already been discussed, and as it was well ascertained that two-thirds of the poor were being robbed, and the other third poisoned by adulteration, he thought it was high time the measure was proceeded with. The adjournment of the debate was moved by Mr Stapleton..."

Time then ran out. The second reading was adjourned for six days, then postponed again on no less than three occasions between March and May. On May 26, an angry Mr Muntz wrote to John Postgate as follows.

> "I withdrew the bill last night, as there is no chance of its coming on again this session: next session we must begin earlier. [In the context of a different debate a few days ahead] I hope that I may have a chance [of] shewing up

> the fallacy that "Free Trade" requires that people should not be prevented from poisoning and plundering wholesale."

In the interval Postgate invited Muntz to his house and demonstrated adulteration, including some sherry which actually had sulphuric acid in it, arranging for suitable publicity in the local and London press. Muntz re-introduced the bill in February of 1871 and again it passed its first reading easily. This time it got through its second reading, discussion being postponed to the committee stage and, after a hitch in April when the House was counted out, the House went into committee and it was actually discussed late in May. It met with opposition as usual, survived an amendment by its opponents to postpone the discussion for six months, but then another parliamentary trick was employed: an opponent moved to "report progress", which effectively meant that the matter went into abeyance. This was agreed. The parliamentary session was due to end before there was any chance of discussion being resumed; Muntz could only withdraw the bill, which he did on 1 June. However, he was optimistic; in a letter to Postgate next day he wrote:

> "I was compelled to retire the bill at 1 o'clock, it being opposed ... We have however, made progress and shall have a fair chance next year. If you still have a copy of your *original* bill, I should be glad if you would let me have it next August, I have mislaid mine."

The original bill was quite a strong one, and Muntz approved of it. He planned to introduce it early in the next year, so, on 3 February, 1872, Postgate held yet another meeting at his home, with suitable press publicity, to demonstrate, using numerous freshly-purchased samples obtained locally, that the adulteration of food, drinks and drugs was as bad as it had been before the Act of 1860 had been passed. Ten days later, on 13 February, Muntz introduced the original bill brought up to date to include the provisions of the Act of 1860 and another relevant Act, the Pharmacy Act of 1868. It passed its first reading uneventfully. However, on its second reading it clearly overlapped with another bill, the Government Public Health Bill. This presented a tricky situation which the adulteration bill's opponents could have exploited; Muntz succeeded in persuading parliament to agree its second reading on the understanding that, if the Public Health bill were passed, his bill would be withdrawn at its third reading. In the event, the Government withdrew the clauses dealing with adulteration from its public health bill. Muntz's bill reached its third reading on 3 July and the House moved into committee to debate it in detail. Half way through the proceedings, an opponent again moved to report progress –

admitting that he had never read the bill! This time all was not lost but its future was in the balance. Langford [6.15] gave the following nail-biting abstract of its parliamentary history:

> "July 9, Bill down again for committee. House counted out at 9 o'clock, just after it re-assembled. July 11, Bill passed through the Committee, at half-past 2 a.m., on the 12th, with amendments. July 15, Report considered at 2 a.m. on the 16th. July 22nd, Bill passed, being read a third time, at ten minutes to 2 a.m., Thursday morning, July 23rd. July 23rd, Bill brought into the House of Lords by Lord Salisbury. Read a first time and ordered to be printed. July 26, Bill read a second time. July 29, Bill passed through committee. July 30, Report of amendments considered and agreed to. August 1, Bill read a third time, and passed in the House of Lords. August 3rd, on motion of Mr Muntz, the Lords amendments were considered and agreed to by the House of Commons. House of Lords, August 6, the Commons amendments to the bill were considered and agreed to. August 10th, the Royal Assent was given to the Bill, and it became law."

Thus, after another three bills, amounting to ten in all, an Act which included effectively everything John Postgate had asked for in 1854 became law – in 1872.

The passage of the bill through the Lords was greatly helped by Lord Eustace Cecil, who urged the Government to support the bill and prompted Lord Salisbury with amendments to increase its stringency at the committee stage. (Lord Eustace had been approached and briefed by Postgate in the Spring of that year.) And to paraphrase Langford [6.16], it was the "skilful pilotage" of Mr Muntz which conducted it successfully through the Commons. At the root of it all, however, was John Postgate's energy and single-mindedness – and, of course, Victorian parliamentary democracy, however lumbering, creaky and slow it might be.

Postgate's work was not quite over. In practice the 1872 Act proved to have flaws and ambiguities. Postgate wrote advice to authorities whenever he became aware of a difficulty. A major problem stemmed from the Act's definition of what constituted adulteration: "any article of food or drink or any drug mixed with any other substances, with intent fraudulently to increase its weight or bulk, without declaration of such admixture to any purchaser thereof before delivering the same." Colouring or flavouring agents, which might have no detectable effect on weight or bulk, seemed to be excluded, though some of these were notoriously toxic. A second important problem, which had applied to all previous Acts, too, was that 'intent' could be difficult to establish in law, especially in cases of imported materials such as tea, where adulteration was sometimes practised abroad, by the manufacturer or exporter. The Act was working. Cases of adulteration of both food and drugs were in decline. A network of Public Analysts had been established and the Society of Public Analysts, formed in 1874 in response to its passage, was set to become an influential body, both scientifically and socially. But magistrates interpreted the Act differently in different parts of the country and the situation generated many complaints, tea dealers being especially vociferous. In 1874 the House of Commons set up a Committee to enquire into its workings [6.17].

The Committee, which included Mr Muntz, found that it had a great deal of work to do and spent many days taking evidence, much of it from aggrieved parties. Hassall was called, and confirmed his earlier views, though he acknowledged that his active interest in problems of adulteration had largely ceased. Postgate was not called. The Committee's problems do not need to be described in detail here, though a bizarre situation regarding tea is worth mentioning. Mr Whitworth Jackson, a London tea wholesaler, gave detailed evidence of tea adulteration as practised by tea dealers, during which, by passing a magnet over a glass tube containing orange Pekoe tea, he demonstrated that it had been adulterated with gummed clusters of iron filings [6.18]. This was but one of his alleged adulterations; others included addition of dried, spent tea leaves, of quartz particles to add weight, of dyes and astringents. A fortnight later, his uncle and father, William and Robert Jackson, both London dealers, appeared before the Committee to refute Whitworth Jackson's allegations angrily, claiming that Whitworth had effectively accused them of adulterations, his uncle describing Whitworth's allegations as imaginary [6.19]. Whitworth was re-examined and maintained his position, but sufficient doubt had been cast for the Committee to regard his evidence as unsafe. Nevertheless, the Committee found that adulteration, though on the decrease, was still widespread, but that the Act was leading to injustice and needed clarification. In the same year Postgate sent a letter to Parliament's Local Government Board proposing a dozen amendments of detail to the 1872 Act which would clarify and improve the Act. These were mainly adopted next year, becoming part of the Sales of Food & Drugs Act of 1875 – which wisely avoided using the word adulteration altogether. It also side-stepped the issue of intent by requiring the accused to show that he or she not only knew nothing of the adulteration detected, but "could not with reasonable diligence have obtained that knowledge." In the same year the Public Health Act 1875, which initiated universal sanitation, was passed, the two Acts making it a year of great significance in the history of public health in Britain.

The 1875 Adulteration Act worked, and it remained in force until 1928, when it formed part of a consolidated Food and Drugs (Adulteration) Act. Only minor abuses, such as misleading claims on packaged foods, continued to slip through the net until, in 1940, the Ministry of Food was granted wider powers which, in essence, still operate. Revisions and devolution leading to separate Acts for Scotland and Northern Ireland in the 1950s [6.20] do not alter the position that John Postgate's Act of 1875 remains the basis of to-day's legislation.

Chapter 7

"JOHN THE DOCTOR"

What kind of person was this John Postgate? (His grandchildren used to refer to him as "John the Doctor", and that name for him persists in the family to this day.)

To be a doctor in Victorian times was indeed something special. Despite the conservatism and nepotism, as well as the occasional fraud and quackery, which had led Wakley to found *The Lancet*, doctors were revered. Advances in medical treatment, initiated by Jenner's spectacular successes with vaccination against smallpox at the turn of the century, had rendered doctors, at least the younger ones, paragons of virtue in the public eye. They were widely expected to be men (but never women) of learning and moral integrity, public-spirited, dedicated to the well-being of their patients and to the integrity of their profession. The upright, reforming Dr Lydgate, hero of George Eliot's *Middlemarch* (1872), perhaps epitomised their mid-century image: a man who combined practice with research and whose innovations brought him into conflict with the establishment, as well as with old-fashioned, more conservative doctors. It would have come as no surprise to the public that Wakley, Hassall, Postgate and many of the witnesses who came before Scholefield's Committee of Enquiry were doctors of one kind or another. Even Charles Kingsley had had medical training.

In outline, John Postgate conformed to the stereotype of his era. He was a self-made success. He had risen by his own efforts from poor, artisan origins to acclaimed professional achievement: a Professor, surgeon and social reformer. Through his writings and his verbatim evidence to the Scholefield Committee, one glimpses an austere, almost forbidding, figure: high principled and proud, somewhat humourless, much concerned for the poor, immensely energetic, and above all determined to right perceived wrongs. It took him twenty-one years – 1854 to 1875 – of dogged lobbying, cajoling and persuading, as well as pamphleteering, lecturing and demonstrating, to obtain an Act of Parliament which he could regard as reasonably satisfactory. It is an image that is not inconsistent with his portrait, painted by Vivian Crome in 1878, which still hangs in a committee room of the Scarborough Town Hall [7.1]. Darkened with age though it is, and poorly hung for lighting, one can yet see him, tight-lipped, of ascetic aspect, fixing the viewer with a stern but distant gaze. He is in academic robes, possibly lecturing, because his left hand is gesturing; in the background one can faintly discern a pestle and mortar, and he holds in his right hand a vessel which is probably a laboratory vial, charged with something rather nasty.

Was his stubborness part of a Postgate heritage, shared by Father Nicholas perhaps? It is certainly not uncommon among his descendents, though that is another story. It is hardly a recipe for widespread popularity. On one occasion the windows of Postgate's house at 41 Frederick Street, to which he had moved from Belmont Place, were deliberately broken, and on another he was shot at; a biographical sketch of his life [7.2] written in 1880 records also that he was offered "testimonials" (probably a euphemism for bribes) if he would desist from his campaign. "Neither offers nor threats, however, turned him from his purpose."

No record or hint remains of how good a medical practitioner he was, how easy he was with his patients, how effective were his treatments. One can only guess that he was austere, confident, deeply concerned for his patients' well-being – particularly that of his poorer patients – but perhaps unlikely to have been more than minimally amiable or patient himself.

Some indications exist bearing upon his personality as an academic. He certainly inspired respect among his colleagues, and his lectures at Sydenham College were a success. The College Principal, physician Dr Bell Fletcher, supported his campaign against drug adulteration, and early in 1855 Postgate

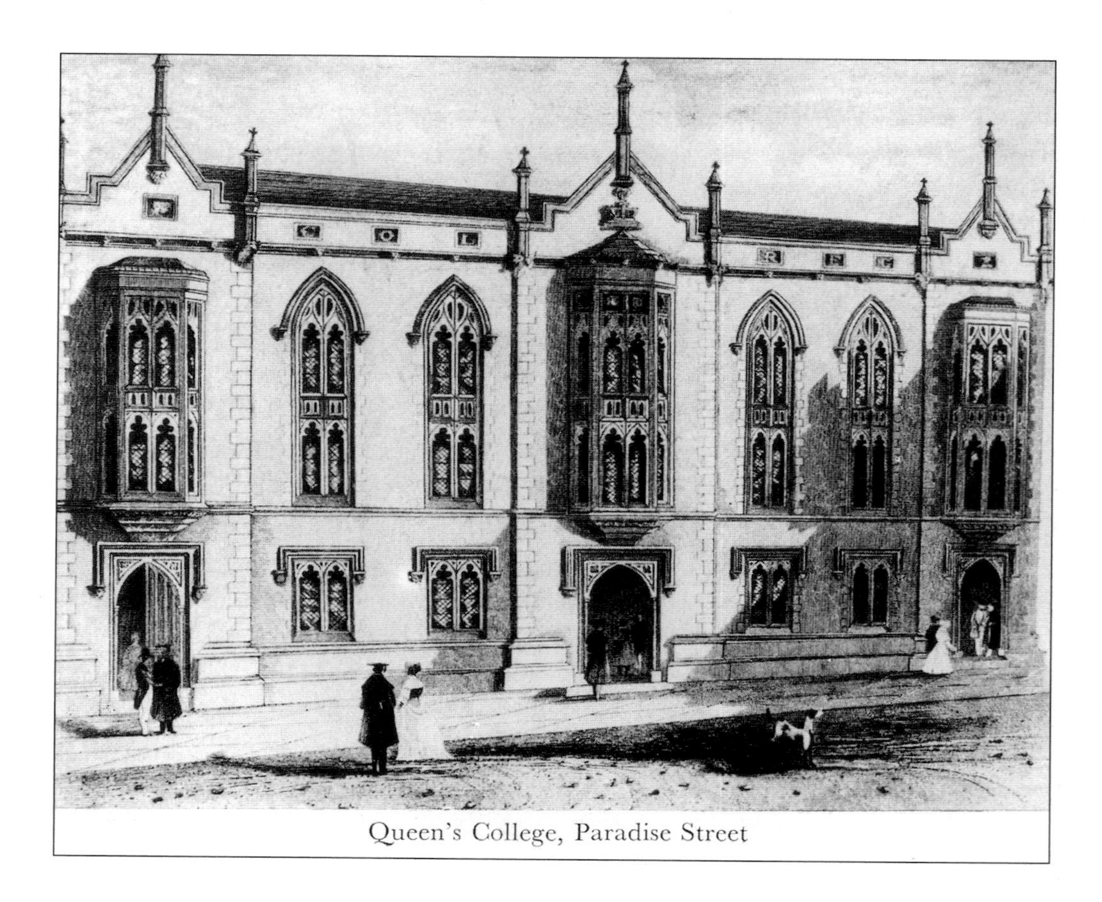

Queen's College, Paradise Street

passed his original subject of anatomy to another teacher and gave lectures on forensic medicine instead. How long he remained on the staff of Sydenham College is not clear; however, as I have recounted in Chapter 6, on 7 May 1860 he was appointed Professor of Medical Jurisprudence and Toxicology at Queen's College (Sydenham's rival) where he remained, lecturing in both the medical and the law departments, for many years. Queen's College's problems with Dr Sands Cox, which had prompted the foundation of Sydenham College several years earlier (see ref. 3.8) had not been wholly resolved, but Postgate soon became a respected figure in the college and was able to assist in its management in various ways. He served as Treasurer of the medical faculty, evincing, in his own words [7.3], "humble prudence, with a somewhat old-fashioned horror of debt." The Professoriate elected him as their representative on the College Council.

In 1862 the Council asked him to give the introductory address to the new intake of medical students, and the text was published a decade or so later [7.4]. Although his welcoming talk would seem, to a twenty-first-century student, hortatory, prescriptive and humourless – 'stuffy' would sum it up – that was the manner of the period and, read with sympathy, it is very perceptive. While surveying the broad academic and professional prospects ahead of his young audience, it illuminates his own philosophical outlook on medicine and Victorian society.

It starts with a list of the qualities of character required in a student of medicine, which might almost serve as a description of himself. The requirements according to Professor Postgate were:

> "1. Good health, without which all thoughts and all efforts are puny, incomplete and inoperative. 2. A well-balanced and evenly-regulated mind. 3. Unselfishness. 4. Fixity of purpose. 5. An unswerving determination to do always what is right, let the consequences be what they may. 6. Clearness of perception. 7. Promptness of action. 8. General benevolence; and, I may add, 9. General contempt for the luxuries and comforts of life, looking for reward to that satisfaction, peace, and contentment of conscience, which flows from the conviction of human misery alleviated, and of human life prolonged, by duties faithfully discharged and services cheerfully rendered."

(One must remember that mid-nineteenth-century medical students were not much different from to-day's, and the temptations to escape from the rigours of academe were just as plentiful: parties, balls, drinking, song, gambling; music hall rather than cinema or theatre, perhaps, and carriages and horses rather than fast cars. The austerity of his catalogue of virtues was probably salutary.)

After exhorting his audience to attentiveness, industry, note-taking at lectures etc., he continued by bringing out the primacy of anatomy in their course, the importance of chemistry and pharmacy, the immediacy of physiology – and offered botany as something of a relief amongst their labours. In the context of chemistry and pharmacy, he could not resist introducing food and drug adulteration, but he restricted his scope to its relevance to medical practice, and made a new, non-political point about his plans: that a network of public analysts would lead to advances in the underlying science. Then he turned to the professional prospects of his students, once they had passed their examinations. Here his message was far from bland. The profession was not a short cut to wealth. Much of the demand for medical help would come from the poor, but Poor-Law surgeons were grossly under-financed by the Poor-Law Guardians and the poor suffered accordingly. He even went so far as to ask, rhetorically, whether the Poor-Law surgeons ought to strike on behalf of their patients. He criticised clubs which sold tickets for medical relief from self-supporting dispensaries: these degraded the profession. He expressed his objection to the manner in which public medical officers were chosen; he inveighed against the willingness of doctors to go to court and give evidence against each other in cases where patients sued for negligence (the current situation in the USA is not new!). His account of the profession was far from starry-eyed as he averred that it was afflicted with "many evils", but he ended on an uplifting note: he had great hopes that the recently established General Medical Council would bring to the profession a status "commensurate with the advantages and benefits it confers on the community".

In conclusion he alluded to the recent administrative troubles that the College had gone through, which everyone would have known about, and made a tactful comment on the virtues of the College's founder, Sands Cox.

The indignation which he expressed in his talk about the pay of Poor-Law surgeons reveals another aspect of his concern for the impoverished. In 1862 he published a pamphlet entitled *Medical Services and Public Payments* [7.5]. This was cited in his entry in the *Dictionary of National Biography*, but all copies seem to have vanished. It is likely that his remarks to the medical freshmen expressed his thesis, that inadequate pay was leading to inadequate medical services, which was bringing the profession into disrepute. The loss of the pamphlet is regrettable because, being John Postgate, he would surely have proposed remedies, probably in considerable detail.

Postgate was nothing if not self-assured and confident of the rightness of his opinions on medical matters. In other areas, too, his views seem to have been firmly held, and though there is no evidence that he was especially religious, he was a firmly Protestant Christian. The story is told among his descendents that a young Catholic priest, hoping to enlist John the Doctor's support for the canonisation of Father Nicholas, called upon him in Birmingham, bringing some holy relics including, according to Postgate's grandson Raymond Postgate [7.6],

> "... a severed finger and a handkerchief stained with the blood of the martyr ..... Grandfather was so indignant at being approached by this young man that he leapt from his desk and tried to seize the idolatrous relics from him. There was a short and unedifying struggle between the two; but the priest was a younger man and he escaped with the relics in his hand and was pursued by the enthusiastic doctor who was too short-winded to catch up with him."

But is that story to be believed? Raymond's generation of Postgates certainly accepted it, but the episode appears in a quite different and more dignified form in the 1880 sketch of John Postgate's life mentioned earlier [7.7]. It records that, at the height of his campaign against adulteration:

> "... he received an invitation from a priest, and in consequence called at the Roman Catholic Church in Birmingham, when his correspondent, after congratulating him on his labours, remarked that the spirit of martyrdom was still in the family, and that he would show him something which would prove of great interest. The priest left the room, but soon returned with a box full of relics, from which he carefully took a piece of coarse linen, in which were some grey hairs. The linen had stains on it, and turning to Mr Postgate, the priest said, "This is the blood of your family 200 years old. This is the blood of Father Nicholas. The linen was part of his shirt, and the hairs were cut from his head after his execution at York." He then offered Mr Postgate the relics, who at once politely refused, "Put them up, my good sir. they will be of more use to you than to me ..."

Yet would a Roman Catholic priest have offered such relics, so precious to his church, to a Protestant. and one who could at best be but a distant relative of the martyr? However, there is internal evidence that the biographical sketch was based on an interview with Postgate himself, so that rendering of the story, be it correct or sanitised, must be the authorised version.

John Postgate's image as a family man is very difficult to establish. His obsessiveness undoubtedly spoiled his relations with his immediate family. It seems clear that he extended the ninth of his prerequisites of a good medical man – "general contempt for the luxuries and comforts of life" – to his whole family, and several of his offspring, perhaps all of them, came to dislike him very much. For one thing, all his politicking for the Adulteration Acts cost money: travel, pamphlets, postage and even samples for analysis had to be paid for, and Postgate paid out of his own income. Though he expected, and received, credit and approval from the right-minded public for his efforts on their behalf, financial recognition was not part of his expectations, and he received none.

A practising doctor, an FRCS who later also became a Professor was in one of Victorian society's upper income brackets and could expect to be comfortably wealthy. Because of his campaign Postgate never became so. He moved house in Birmingham three times [7.8], and that must have cost a great deal, but he devoted almost all of his income to his cause. His wife Mary Ann, as will be discussed later, bore the brunt of his sacrifices for the community, for she was always short of money for essentials needed to feed, clothe and generally look after the large family. Equally the children grew up to resent their parsimonious and uncaring father. Postgate's grandson Raymond was told by his father, John Percival, that 'John the Doctor' "was so devoted to the cause of preventing adulteration that he used to steal from grandmother's purse the money which he had given to her already for house-keeping, in order to spend it on pamphlets." That John the Doctor took a cavalier view of any money possessed by his wife is confirmed by a letter John Percival wrote to Raymond in 1923:

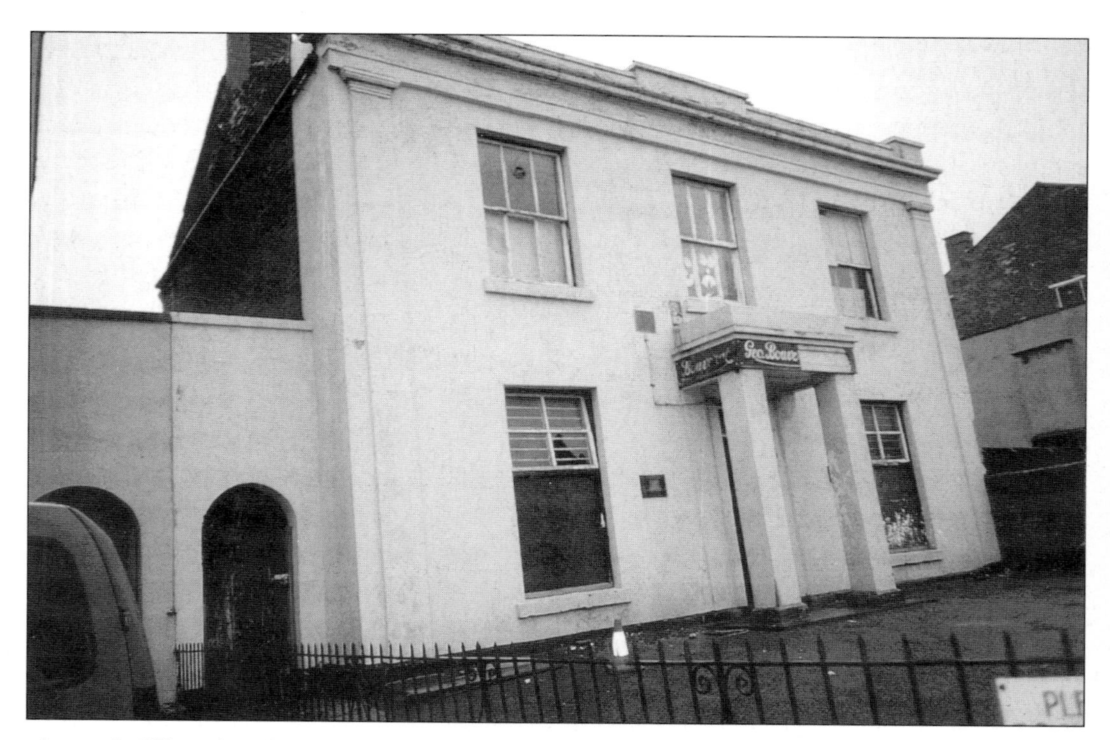

An early Victorian house in Frederick Street in 1998. Postgate's residence, number 41, had been demolished.

"Amongst the things which your grandmother treasured was a five guinea piece of George II issued in the early part of his reign. A very great many years ago while your grandfather was still alive she gave it into my charge as she feared that he might sell it and appropriate the proceeds. I placed it with my bankers for safe custody ...."

John Percival also told Raymond that two of his sisters were so underfed because of John the Doctor's meanness that at "the age of fourteen they went mad". Whether their derangement was due to inadequate food, family stress, or some other cause, it is certainly true that Agnes Foord and the second Mary Ann were mentally unstable and spent the last twenty years of their lives incapacitated in asylums, their affairs being managed by a relative. They died within days of each other in 1920. How far John the Doctor can be held responsible for their conditions is not clear: John Percival clearly had a low opinion of his father and was a prejudiced witness. But other Postgates of Raymond's generation have confirmed that John Postgate's family suffered for his cause.

Isabella Jane, the eldest daughter, liked to be known as Isa. She was not mad, but she certainly became somewhat eccentric [7.9]. And she shared her siblings' dislike of their father. In a booklet entitled *A Trilogy of Victorian Saints*, published in 1930 [7.10] (dedicated to her clergyman brother Langdale Postgate), she wrote about the saintly lives of her mother, her paternal grandmother (Harriett Horwood, referred to in the booklet as "Your dear Granny") and Harriett's companion Edna ("A Faithful Handmaiden"). Her mother was thinly disguised – it is not clear why – under the pseudonym "The Rose of Flatfield". (Flatfield is where Isa placed the home of "Your dear Granny". There is no such community in the Oxford University Press's Gazetteer of Britain [7.11] and it may be a pseudonym for Driffield, the Horwoods' home town.)

Her chapter on Harriett gives an evocative glimpse of her brothers John (Lionel) and Langdale dressed to visit "Your dear Granny" with their mother:

> "... The two young scamps, so spruce and proud in their grey tunics with glossy patent leather belts and serpent-shaped clasps, and black velvet peaked caps on their bonny little heads..."

However, it is her chapter on her mother which best reveals her opinion of her father. Of Mary Ann's marriage to John Postgate she wrote:

> "...It is sad to record that, with all her charms and chances, poor Rose [Mary Ann] did in the end pick up a very crooked stick; and her life, so full of promise, darkened into a long tragedy. She was then indeed transplanted into

an arid soil, and drab and dead was the atmosphere around her. Straightened means, a large young family and unceasing domestic cares and toil left no room for literary efforts..."

That chapter includes a poetic account of the death of the first Mary Ann, her mother's first-born daughter, who lived for less than two years. Its general message is that her mother's faith in God sustained her throughout a life of dreadful impositions, and Isa's own feelings about her father are made abundantly clear:

> "Throughout much crushing sorrow and years of well-nigh unbearable bondage the Rose kept her bright spirit and bravely did her duty as a faithful wife, and a most devoted, loving mother. In spite of what was often real and trying persecution she retained her firm, simple trust in God and never swerved from her strong religious principles."

Mary Ann did indeed love her children and looked after them as best she could. She lived to the age of 83, surviving her husband by seven years, and though in later life she was much troubled by arthritis she remained an energetic, rather formidable person. Margaret (later Dame Margaret) Cole, daughter of John Percival Postgate, remembered in her autobiography [7.12] a visit to her grandmother shortly before her death in 1898:

> "....she was either wholly or partly bedridden. I remember being taken to see her in her big bed, a grim old lady with a cap and a nose and by her side a parrot in a cage (with much the same kind of nose) which squawked out menacingly, "Maar-*gret*! Maar-*gret*!" when I came near. I was terrified of both the parrot and my grandmother ..."

Margaret also remembered being told that her grandparents were always quarrelling.

John Postgate sired seven children in all. John Percival, who was known as Percy in the family, inherited his father's bent for teaching, though in the wholly different area of the Classics. A scholar of Trinity College, Cambridge, he took a distinguished degree and was quickly elected to a Fellowship; he later became Professor of Comparative Philology at University College, London, and, finally, Professor of Latin at Liverpool University [7.13]. Like his father, he felt he had a mission: in his case it was to reform the teaching and pronunciation of Latin [7.14]; again like his father, he aroused the antagonism of his own children [7.15]. The second child (the first infant to bear the name Mary Ann) died young, as has been mentioned. Isabella Jane, too, we have met; did her religious writings echo her mother's Christianity and literary aspirations? Of Agnes Foord Postgate and the second Mary Ann nothing is recorded beyond John Percival's statement (p.65) that both were mentally unstable. The doctor's fifth offspring and his namesake, John, was nicknamed Lionel, presumably to avoid confusion in the family's day-to day activities. He died tragically, drowned in the river Cherwell, while an undergraduate reading Classics at Oxford; his literary memorial is a volume of translations of Latin poetry [7.16]. Langdale Horwood Postgate became a Church of England clergyman, for some 35 years vicar of All Saints, Shillington, in Bedfordshire. He also became a Canon of St Albans. He was another remarkable character; he and his benefactions to the church are still remembered in that community [7.17]. The re-use of the name Mary Ann and the choice of the name John for two of their sons by John the Doctor and his wife seem to denote a desire to perpetuate their own names in the next generation. A feature of his will, however, suggests that his sons were reluctant to co-operate in this. He drew up his will in May of 1878 – more of its details later – and in March of 1879 he added a curious codicil requiring his sons to retain their names and initials unaltered, or else forfeit their portion of his estate, receiving in its place one shilling. This clearly reflected some kind of domestic *contretemps* in which one or more of his sons wished to change their name(s). Could it be that Lionel, whose only given name was John, and who was so named for his father, wished to change to his nickname? Was the codicil a threat to cut him off with a shilling if he did so? If so, he and his father reached some kind of a *rapprochement*, for in a later, undated, codicil, his father specifically excluded John (Lionel), together with Mary Ann jnr, from that provision.

The will as a whole was fairly conventional for its period. His estate and income from stocks and shares went to his three sons, who were to be his executors, with the provision that they "permit and suffer my dear wife Mary Ann Postgate to use and enjoy [his house, belongings etc] for the benefit of all my children and herself during her lifetime free from debt...". The actual monetary income from his investments was to be divided six ways among his three sons and three daughters and, when each reached the age of 65, one sixth of the investments would be sold and the capital realised inherited by the legatee. Thus he treated his "dear wife" rather badly; she inherited no income of her own and her expenses were controlled by her children. After the fuss about names referred to above, it seems he had doubts about his sons' reliability as executors, and in his second codicil he made his daughters executors too. His will does not reflect a man confident of the goodwill of his offspring.

Clearly his family was far from happy. But he himself may have been too detached, too much involved in his work and his campaign to be greatly aware of it. Victorian fathers normally expected, indeed preferred, to be remote, authoritarian figures in their children's eyes; displays of overt concern or affection were regarded as almost unmanly. According to his obituarist in *The Times* [7.18], he loved his children, and was devastated when Lionel, to whom he was said to have been "devotedly attached", was drowned. Even here there is a disquieting overtone of emotional disorder: there has always been a suggestion within the family, but nothing more than a suggestion, that Lionel's death was suicide rather than an accident.

John Postgate's inflexible principles and priorities made him put the good of his fellows above the needs of his family. Therefore, though his public persona as an academic and a splendid Victorian reformer is reasonably clear, his personality as a family man and parent is shadowy, distorted by hostile recollections. Yet how could a character so unpleasant as Isa depicted have retained the friendship and goodwill of Scholefield, Muntz, his fellow academics and his many supporters among Birmingham's citizens? The truth must lie somewhere between those family recollections and the admiration expressed by Langford, by his anonymous biographer for *The Biograph & Review*, and by his obituarists: a man easy to admire but difficult to love.

Postgate lived long enough to see the fruits of his labours, as the 1875 Act began to take effect. By the late 1870s he had begun to suffer from digestive disorders. These became increasingly distressing and painful – perhaps that is why he made a will – and, in 1881, accompanied by a daughter, he visited Neuenahr in Germany to take a cure. On his return journey he was suddenly taken very ill while crossing London. At his own request he was taken to the London Hospital, where he had once been a student; he died of a stomach cancer on the day of his admission: 26 September 1881 [7.19]. His estate was valued at £6678.18s.10d.

He was buried in Birmingham's 'new cemetery' [7.20]. His epitaph read:

> "For twenty-five years of his life without reward and under heavy discouragement he laboured to protect the health and purify the commerce of this people".

Chapter 8

HIS ACHIEVEMENT

Postgate's fame by the end of his life was such that, of the three prime movers in this story, only he and Wakley were accorded entries in the *Dictionary of National Biography* [8.1, 8.2]; surprisingly, and quite unjustly, Hassall was omitted.

Postgate's obituarist in *The Times* wrote of him:

> "Indeed, it is not too much to say that it is primarily to the scientific skill and benevolent zeal of Mr Postgate that we owe the existing laws against the adulteration of food and drugs."[8.3]

His obituarist in the *British Medical Journal* was factual. He rightly emphasised his professional and financial self-sacrifice, and gave him all credit for the Adulteration Acts [8.4].

His anonymous biographer in *The Biograph & Review* had concluded his account with a positively rhapsodic assessment of his achievement:

> "It was a great work, achieved against terrible odds, which only the deepest faith, the most earnest zeal, indomitable courage could overcome. Mr Postgate has displayed all these virtues, has overcome all the difficulties, and deserves all the honours which are due to such a victory."[8.5]

Widely known, much admired and sometimes feared in his day, John Postgate's name has now all but vanished from the history books [8.6]. Why is this? The probable reasons, only partly of his own making, are less than edifying.

The eulogies above reflect how Postgate's political influence and public fame had grown as his crusade, as the *British Medical Journal* termed it, progressed. In the public eye, he had effectively taken over from Wakley and Hassall who, whether justly or not, must have seemed content simply to expose instances of fraud and adulteration and hope that the legislature would do something. That Postgate adopted the issue, and proposed (and ultimately obtained) effective remedies, ought to have been a source of satisfaction and collaboration all round.

For a brief period, perhaps it was. In 1854 *The Lancet* published the circular letter of Postgate and Browne to the medical profession (p.32). But very soon Wakley and Hassall must have noticed a striking feature of Postgate's writings, letters and reported evidence: that their names were not once mentioned. On only one occasion for which Postgate was responsible – the resolution passed by the Birmingham meeting of April 1854 (p.32) – were the efforts of *The Lancet* acknowledged. Even in his evidence to the Scholefield Committee, Postgate attributed his original interest in adulteration to a patient who had been made ill by drinking adulterated coffee, not to *The Lancet*'s exposures, though he cannot have been unaware of them. And he kept up his indifference: the biographical sketch of 1880 mentioned above, over which he must have had considerable influence, made no mention of the *The Lancet*'s team.

This disregard of fellow contributors cannot be excused. Postgate may have learned about adulteration independently of Wakley and Hassall, first as a grocer's boy, then as a dispensary assistant, but he can hardly have been unaware of the tremendous contribution made by *The Lancet*'s Analytical Commission, and if by some remarkable oversight he only learned of it in 1854, he ought to have acknowledged it publicly in his later writings.

His public attitude to their work must have been vexing to the pioneers, the more so as this young upstart's fame and influence grew. Certainly *The Times*'s enthusiasm in his obituary, especially the passage quoted above, contrasted markedly with The Lancet's brief note of his death [8.7]. It also provoked a resentful riposte [8.8] in a subsequent issue of *The Lancet* written by Dr James Wakley, Thomas's son, who was by then its editor. He pointed out, reasonably enough, that John Postgate had simply built upon the earlier work of their own Commission and that Hassall was the Scholefield Committee's principal and most authoritative witness. No doubt similar thinking prompted Wakley's biographer, writing in 1897, to make no mention at all of John Postgate, even in a chapter devoted to food and drug adulteration and the Acts [8.9]. He disregarded Postgate's activities, both analytical and political, and attributed the setting up of the Scholefield Committee of Enquiry, and the passage of the Adulteration Acts of 1860, 1872 and 1875, entirely to Wakley and Hassall, as stemming from *The Lancet*'s reports of the findings of its Analytical Commission.

It must have been a deliberate omission, for the biographer cannot have been unaware of the part Postgate had played. But antagonisms were indeed rife among the reformers involved with adulteration and Postgate was far from the only one to be subject to, and guilty of, ungallant behaviour. Professor Redwood, whose evidence to Scholefield's Committee was balanced and reasonable, not seriously in conflict with Hassall's actual findings, was nevertheless a severe critic of Hassall's claims and views. And to put the point mildly, Hassall's recollections of his own achievements appear sometimes to have been over-subjective and dismissive of others [8.10]. A short-lived rift between Hassall and Wakley was mentioned on p.29; at the time, July – August 1855, a serious controversy developed in the correspondence columns of *The Times*, initiated by Hassall's claiming credit for inspiring both *The Lancet*'s Analytical Commission and Scholefield's Enquiry; he also down-graded Letheby's contribution to the Commission's analytical work. Both Wakley and Letheby reacted with annoyance. Wakley objected to his earlier efforts with O'Shaugnessy and others being set aside; Letheby gave details of the many chemical analyses, and advice on procedures, that he had provided for Hassall: some 290 analyses for *The Lancet*'s Commission (Hassall claimed to have performed 2197 mainly microscopical analyses). *The Lancet* reproduced the correspondence substantially unabridged [8.11]; in it, one (anonymous) correspondent mentioned Postgate's role in calling the Birmingham meeting. *The Lancet*'s reprinting was preceded by an editorial comment emphasising Wakley's role and acknowledging Letheby's contribution, the scale of which *The Lancet* – presumably meaning Wakley himself – claimed not to have known. The rift did not last. Hassall and Wakley were reconciled, superficially at least, by the time of the testimonial dinner for Hassall (p.29), which was held in the Spring of 1856: Wakley, replying to a toast proposed by Hassall, referred to their differences as, "merely a lovers' quarrel and we are now greater friends than ever."[8.12] Dr. Letheby, however, continued to resent not receiving more credit, even though his part was subsidiary rather than major. He later wrote the article on adulteration for the 9th edition of the *Encyclopædia Britannica* (1875) in which, rather childishly, he made no mention at all of Hassall's work, but cited his own [8.13]. The eleventh through to the fourteenth editions cited both Hassall and Wakley, and Letheby was dropped out; none mentioned Postgate.

In this connection Hassall's obituary in *The Lancet* is a remarkable document. Writing in 1894, his obituarist departed from the well-established Victorian convention of *de mortuis nil nisi bonum* and, "reluctantly" alluding to "some extravagant claims" made by Hassall before Scholefield's Committee, he apportioned credit for action leading to the setting-up of that Committee reasonably fairly among Hassall, his draughtsman Mr Miller, Wakley, Letheby and Postgate [8.14]. However, he wrote only of the mid 1850s, the period of the controversy in correspondence columns of *The Times*, and he concluded his relevant passage with a quotation from *The Lancet*'s editorial bearing upon those letters: that the benefits resulting from its Commission's work were of "too much public importance to allow of their being frittered down to mere questions of individual claims and disputes."

Nevertheless, as far as subsequent developments are concerned, the antagonisms and disputes which arose in the 1850s outlasted all protagonists. Absurdly, they are still reflected in recent histories. Thus Whittet in 1960 [8.15] listed seven twentieth-century standard works dealing with adulteration which omitted all mention of Postgate. Gray [8.16] in his 1983 biography of Hassall made but one reference to Postgate, in a minor context, and got his name wrong. Beeston in 1953, significantly writing from the USA [8.17] had written a corrective article, and both Whittet and Beeston were reproached by Steib in 1966 [8.18] for over-rating Postgate's contribution. However Steib's history was balanced and better informed than most modern accounts. Happily, Burnett's wide-ranging history of 1989 [8.19] also gave a balanced, albeit brief, account of all three protagonists.

To take a generous view of the matter, Postgate was clearly insensitive to the feelings of others in his family life; it is very likely that his self-absorption in this respect spilled over into his political life. Obsessive doers are usually "steamrollers", rarely sensitive to other people's feelings. He was working in parallel with two other obsessives, and such personalities, once they have been offended, remain so; they are also especially susceptible to jealousies.

However, at this distance in time the question of who annoyed or offended the other first no longer matters. A balanced view ought to prevail. For it is clear that, in the political and social context of Victorian England, all three deserve substantial, and probably equal, credit for the really crucial event: the passage of the Act of 1875. Credit is due to Wakley for giving the scandal of adulteration a very courageous kind of publicity – it is difficult to imagine in the 2000s how *The Lancet* was hated in some quarters – and for having the wit to recruit Hassall to his Commission; to Hassall for tackling the problem systematically, so as to build up an irrefutable body of damning evidence; and to Postgate for keeping Hassall's findings before the public, confirming and extending them, and for organising, lobbying, cajoling and briefing politicians, local and national, until a reluctant Government was forced to do something really effective. Given the myriad of issues that demanded reform, and given the deadening opposition Postgate encountered, there can be little doubt that parliament would have procrastinated and delayed indefinitely, had it not been for Postgate's sheer stubbornness. There was without doubt more to the story as a whole, but the eulogies in his obituaries and epitaph, given the constraints of such memorials, were accurate and well-deserved.

ENVOI

At the beginning of this book I remarked how, since the days of the adulteration acts, the food industry had become a huge hi-tech operation with complex routes from harvest to kitchen. Equally the pharmaceutical industry has mushroomed. In both cases the scope for fraud and malpractice became immensely greater. In fact, fraud and malpractice declined so much that today we expect our food to be what it says it is, and to be wholesome and fresh as well; and we expect our medicaments to be trustworthy – at least as far as their composition is concerned.

As a general rule our expectations are justified.

Take food in particular. Considering the number of steps at which something could go wrong in the long chain of processes which bring food to our tables, disasters and misfortunes are rarer than might reasonably be expected. Moreover, when they occur they generate immediate publicity, and officialdom is called to account. In truth, at the start of the new millennium we in the developed countries normally eat remarkably safely; this is true despite occasional outbreaks of food poisoning, as well as the wholly unexpected emergence of BSE towards the end of the twentieth century.

So why, as the twenty-first century begins, do the public and media, in Britain in particular, worry so much about the nature and quality of our food? BSE, of course, had a traumatic effect, and quite rightly so. But fashionable anxieties range far beyond BSE. The most serious is why, despite all we know about hygiene, is the incidence of food poisoning rising? Then there are anxieties about usually manageable risks. Are pesticide or allergenic residues present? Are the additives or preservatives safe? Some worries are to my mind bizarre, such as an undiscriminating objection to genetically engineered crops; yet other worries have little to do with nutrition, quality or taste, but reflect concern over whether the food comes from politically, environmentally or genetically proper sources. However, underlying all these anxieties is our knowledge that the food industry is closely monitored by government. We may worry whether the monitors have got it right, we may doubt government reassurances and object to its prorogations, but if things go wrong we hold the government responsible. Our modern anxieties are the luxuries of a society that expects to be, and normally is, well and wholesomely fed. So we are free to worry about the fine detail.

We owe this freedom, as well as our relative gastronomic and medical security, to the reforming zeal of that formidable trio of Victorians: Thomas Wakely and Arthur Hassall, who publicised their catalogue of abuses, and John Postgate, who doggedly bullied government into doing something about it.

NOTES AND REFERENCES

PREFACE

0.1 John and Mary Postgate, 1994, *A Stomach For Dissent. The Life of Raymond Postgate*. Keele Univ. Press.

0.2 E.W. Steib, 1966, *Drug Adulteration and Control in 19th Century Britain* Madison: U. of Wisconsin Press, USA. (see p.307, note 67). Steib's book is an admirably thorough if occasionally repetitive study of its subject which features all the *dramatis personae* of food adulteration mentioned in the present work, though his emphasis is naturally on medical aspects,

0.3 According to his will, Postgate left his "letters, newspapers and all other miscellaneous documents", plus memorabilia including medals (among them Joshua Horwood's Trafalgar medal – see p.12) and a presentation plate to his son Langdale Horwood. Langdale married, but he had no descendants; he was for many years the vicar of All Saints' church at Shillington in Bedfordshire and a Canon of St Albans. However, my inquiries in the diocese and the parish, in the Postgate family, in the Bedfordshire County Record Office, in the municipal and university libraries of Birmingham, and in the National Register of Archives, yielded no trace of his father's documents.

0.4 J.A. Langford, 1887, *Modern Birmingham and its Institutions*, volumes 1 & 2. Birmingham: William Downing.

0.5 Anon., 1880, John Postgate F.R.C.S. *The Biograph and Review*, (3) (May): 411-417.

0.6 B.T. Davis, 1967, John Postgate. *Birmingham University's Medical Society's Magazine* (a student publication).

CHAPTER 1

1.1 Anon., 1910, Adulteration. *Encyclopædia Britannica* 11th. ed., p.218ff.

1.2 A.J. Amos, (ed.), 1960, *Pure Food and Pure Food Legislation*. London: Butterworth.

1.3 E.W. Steib, 1966, as 0.2, p.136.

1.4 Mrs I. Beeton, 1861, *Book of Household Management*. Facsimile ed., Chancellor Press: London, 1982. pp.671, 831.

1.5 G.D.H. Cole and Raymond Postgate, 1946, *The Common People 1746-1946*. London: Methuen, p. 360.

1.6 John Postgate, 1990, Sticky Breeches and Poisoned Lozenges. *New Scientist* 22/29 December, 31-33.

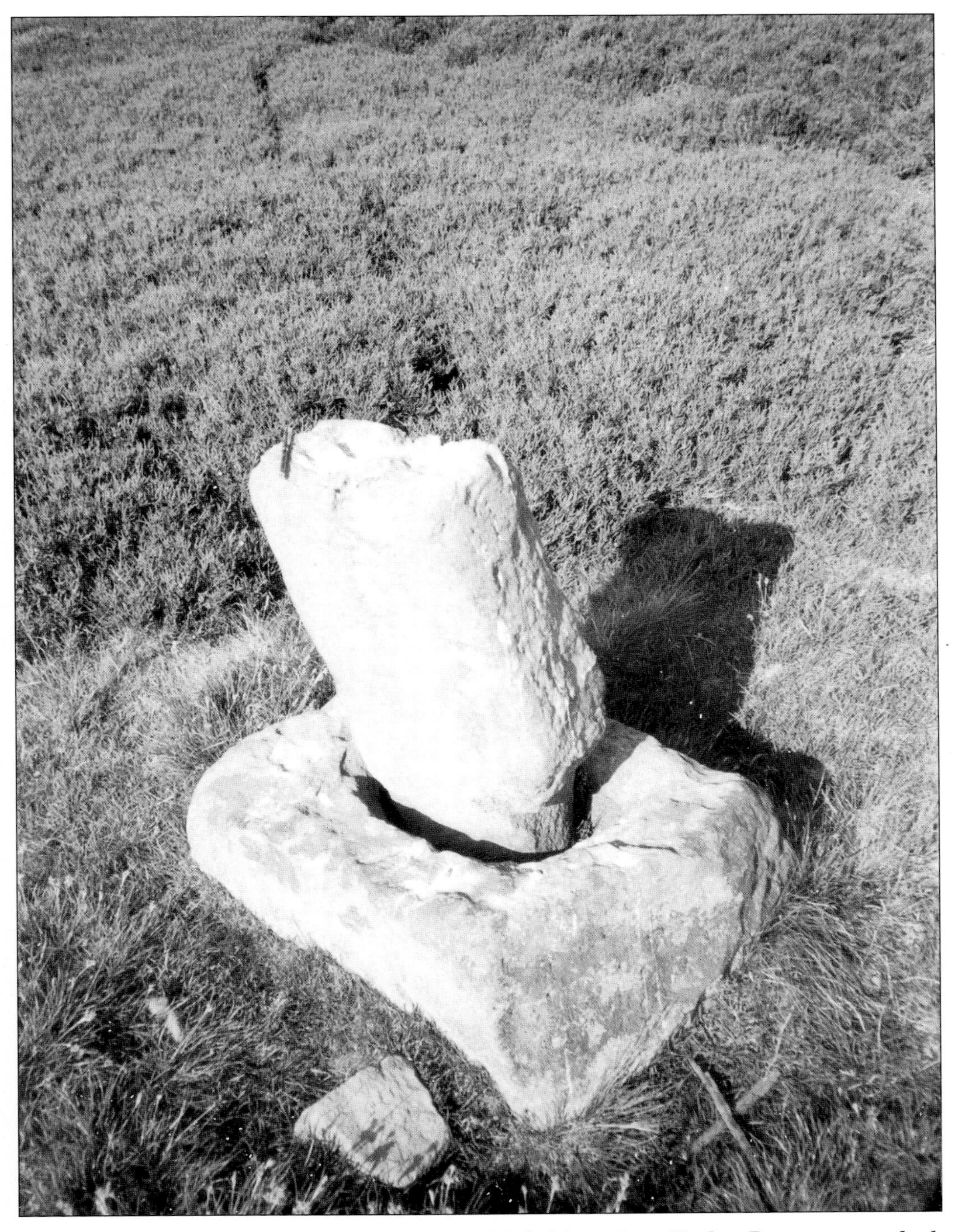

Postgate Cross, on moorland outside Whitby, Yorkshire, where Father Postgate preached. The 'cross' is crudely carved in the flat top of a standing stone; a pen in the photograph indicates the scale.

CHAPTER 2

2.1 Even today the name Postgate is rare outside Yorkshire. There are records from 1200 and 1220 of land in that county being held by Postgates; near Whitby two fields are still known as Upper and Lower Postgate, and Postgate Farm near Glaisdale still exists.

2.2 Nicholas Postgate's martyrdom happened in 1678, during the era of the 'Popish plot'. As a young man he had taken orders in the Roman Catholic church at Douai in France. After nine years he had returned to Yorkshire where, for many years, he had worked as a gardener and, undercover, pursued his vocation as a priest, sometimes using his grandmother's maiden name of Watson as a pseudonym. He was discreet about his religious activities, preaching to his flock at secret places on the Yorkshire moors. Three sheets would be put out as a sign to the faithful that he was due to preach there. One of these secret places still bears his name: a prehistoric stone, marked with a cross, which stands almost hidden from sight at a lonely spot some miles from Whitby is called Postgate Cross. He evaded capture for several decades, possibly because he was a popular figure locally to whom the regional authorities may well have turned a blind eye; the Yorkshire countryside was remote from London, the centre of sectarian conflict, and who could be sure that a new sovereign might not embrace Catholicism again? However, he was ultimately betrayed to the authorities and arrested by one John Reeves, a bitter anti-papist, at Littlebeck while, it is said, baptizing a child into the Roman Catholic church (though the charge against him was simply that of being a Catholic priest). He was tried in 1679 and found guilty. Although by then over 80 years old, he was hanged, drawn and quartered at York. According to *The Victoria History of the Counties of England. A History of Yorkshire North Riding.* 2 p.513. [W Page, ed., 1923, London: St Catherine's Press] Reeves did not benefit from his action: he was drowned with his £20 reward money still in his pocket.

Relics attributed to Father Postgate, including a lock of hair and a signed prayer book, repose in a special shrine in St. Hedda's church at Egton Bridge; even today, once a year in the summer, worshippers fill the church for the "Annual Postgate Rally" to pray for the soul of their local martyr and to hope for his eventual canonization. In 1987 he was beatified by the Vatican and is now correctly designated The Blessed Father Nicholas. [See Roland Connelly, 1987, *No Greater Love. Martyrs of the Middlesborough Diocese.* Gt. Wakering, Essex: McCrimmons; also Elizabeth Hamilton, 1980, *The Priest of the Moors. Reflections on Nicholas Postgate.* London: Darton, Longman & Todd.]

Family tradition also has it that Henry was descended from a Michael Postgate of Great Ayton, a township inland to the North East of Scarborough. Michael founded the Postgate School, where the explorer Captain Cook was

educated; the building still exists, housing an exhibition of Cook *memorabilia*.
2.3 For example, a son of John, John Percival Postgate (later Professor of Latin at Liverpool University), replying to a query from his own son, Raymond (writer and socialist), about their ancestry, remembered:

> "…. 'Uncle Sam' [Samuel Hall Postgate]. He was a publican and a consumer as well as retailer of liquor. He had an eagle – a wretched fowl that he kept in a cage. We were taken to see it on a visit to Scarbro'."

A description wholly consistent with the relaxed, happy gentleman, with poached-egg eyes, depicted in an old sepia photograph dating from 1870-80 which the family still possesses. Samuel Hall kept the Westmount Vaults, later the Carlton Hotel (but still an inn), in the Westborough district of Scarborough. The Carlton was demolished after the Second World War to make room for a new shopping precinct.

Of another uncle, John Percival wrote:

> "'Uncle Tom' [Henry Thomas Postgate] had had an injury to one of his eyes, perhaps received in Australia where he was a gold miner for many years, which gave him a forbidding appearance. When he came back, his mother was his gold mine – he was a regular 'sponger'."

Tom had worked as a joiner before he went to Australia.

William, who became a mariner in the merchant service, married Mary Shires; they had a daughter and a son and the latter, John William Postgate, emigrated to the USA where he pursued a variegated career: he was a newspaper proprietor, a composer of religious poetry and hymns, and a lecturer on tipplers in Shakespeare's plays; among his descendants was Margaret Postgate, a distinguished New York sculptress of the early twentieth century.

Eleanor married Robert Harrowby in 1840 and Rebecca married Richard Wade in 1859. Jane married James Fowler, a mariner, in July of 1866 and the couple emigrated to Canada.

2.4 Untraced; cited by Anon., 1880, as 0.5. Apart from a single issue from 1786, I have been unable to find copies of the *Yorkshire Magazine* dated earlier than 1840.

2.5 Henry Mayhew, 1851, *Mayhew's London* (Edited by Peter Quennell, 1969, London: Spring Books).

2.6 Anon., 1880, as 0.5.

2.7 Thomas Seccombe, 1909, Postgate, John (1820-81). *Dictionary of National Biography*. 16: 203-4. London: Smith, Elder & Co.

2.8 Isa J. Postgate, 1930, *A Trilogy of Victorian Saints*. London: De La More Press.

CHAPTER 3

3.1. Chadwick became to many the most unpopular man in England. One of the principles of the New Poor Law was that the relief offered should be less pleasant than the lowest means of earning a living outside the workhouse, and that the inmates of workhouses should be segregated according to sex, even if they were man and wife, to prevent child-bearing (G.D.H. Cole & Raymond Postgate, 1946, as 1.4, pp. 274-278).

3.2. With the passage of the Public Health Act in 1848 Chadwick became Commissioner of th Government's Board of Health, with the power to instigate local Public Health Boards and to require such surveys.

3.3 C. Gill, 1952, *History of Birmingham* **1**, Oxford U. Press.

3.4 A. Briggs, 1952 *idem* **2**.

3.5 John Postgate, 1852, *The Sanatary Aspect of Birmingham*. Birmingham: Thos. Ragg.

His spelling 'Sanatary' is idiosyncratic if etymologically defensible. 'Sanatory' and the more usual 'sanitary' are both listed (as almost synonymous) in the Oxford English Dictionary; 'sanatary' is not.

3.6 Dale End, Coleshill Street and Great Barr Road were largely built over in the late nineteenth-century reconstruction and are no longer on the town map.

3.7 B.T. Davis, 1967, as 0.6

3.8 Queen's College was founded in 1830, in association with Queen's Hospital, by William Sands Cox FRS. He was an energetic but difficult man, and Sydenham College was founded in association with Birmingham's General Hospital by surgeons and physicians disenchanted with his administration of Queen's. It remained a rival until 1868 when, after radical changes at Queen's (see ref.7.3), the two colleges amalgamated, retaining the name Queen's College Medical School. All but the theological school of Queen's was later assimilated by Mason Science College, which in turn became the nucleus of Birmingham University at its foundation in 1900 (E.W. Vincent & D. Hinton, 1947, *The University of Birmingham. Its History and Significance*. Birmingham: Cornish Brothers).

3.9 See, for example, Stephen Mennell, 1985, *All Manners of Food*. Oxford: Blackwell, pp. 219-220.

3.10 Elizabeth Ray, 1991, *Alexis Soyer, Cook Extraordinary*. Lewes: Southover Press, p.43.

3.11 F. Engels, 1845, *The Condition of the Working Class in England in 1844*. London: Granada, 1969, p.103. Quoted by Mennell, 1985, as 3.9, p.225.

CHAPTER 4

4.1 F.C. Accum, 1820, *Treatise on Adulterations of Food and Culinary Poisons*. London: Longman. Hurst, Rees, Orm & Brown.

4.2 E.W. Steib, 1966, as 0.2, pp.160-169. Accum's entry in the *Dictionary of National Biography* (G.F. Rodwell, 1908, Accum, Friedrich Christian (1769-1838). *Dictionary of National Biography.* **1**:57. London: Smith, Elder & Co.) cannot be relied upon. For example, it described his crime as "embezzlement" and mistook his position at the Royal Institution. Steib's account took in later revisions and was the source of the summary here.
4.3 T.D. Whittet, 1960, Some Contributions of Pharmacy to Pure Food and Drugs. *Chem. & Drugg.* 174:441-2.
4.4 J. Burnett, 1989, *Plenty & Want. A Social History of Food in England from 1815 to the Present day*. 3rd edn. London: Routledge. Chapter 10 of Professor Burnett's comprehensive history comprises an excellent overview of food adulteration in the mid nineteenth century.
4.5 S.S. Sprigge, 1897, *The Life and Times of Thomas Wakley*. London: Longmans, Green & Co.
Wakley came of a large Devonian farming family. His medical training involved apprenticeship to an apothecary, experience and study in London's Borough Hospitals, and specialized study of anatomy. He rapidly became aware of the jobbery and nepotism which were rife among surgeons in the early 1800s and was shocked by the poor quality of medical treatment then available, especially to the poor. Though he spent a few years in private practice, medical reform soon became the principal objective of his life's work, and his periodical *The Lancet* became his most effective weapon in this endeavour. His exposure of the widespread adulteration of food was but one of many issues which he took up, often using unorthodox journalistic methods. *The Lancet*'s reports of teaching surgeons' lectures, thereby exposing their shortcomings as well as making the texts available to a non-paying audience, and its critical reports of bungled or inappropriate hospital operations, incurred the wrath of the medical establishment; some led to legal actions and brought occasional penalties, sometimes nominal because the legislature found itself sympathetic to his side; on at least one occasion his supporters paid his fine by public subscription. Another issue was his concern that seniority and Fellowship of the Royal College of Surgeons should be based on merit, not wealth or family connections, and it was frustration in this endeavour, rather than concern with politics *per se*, that led him to his relatively brief career in parliament – where, however, he became well respected as a spokesman on medical matters.

He was equally a campaigner against medical fraud and for high quality medical service, insisting that medicine should be more 'scientific' – a novel word in those days. He lamented the poor quality of training in anatomy in Britain as compared to France – this against a background of grave-robbing and even murder for medical dissection (as instance the famous Burke and Hare scandals), and he regarded the Anatomy Act of 1832, which he supported, as too weak. He had no time for the then fashionable Mesmerism, which he considered to be largely charlatanry. He regarded vaccination against smallpox as "the greatest boon science ever gave mankind", yet he opposed universal compulsory vaccination, then being mooted, on the grounds (a) that available vaccine preparations were often of poor quality, and (b) that those who would administer the vaccine, especially to the poor, were inadequately trained. Both of these features, he maintained, would bring the treatment into disrepute.

During his life he was best known for his work as a democrat, friend of the poor and Coroner – as in the affair of Thomas Austin. Yet even these activities had a medical basis: he campaigned for good quality, and reasonably paid, medical evidence in court, insisting that medical witnesses and Coroners should be medically qualified. He was astute and, in retrospect, very sound in his many and diverse judgements; history has shown how profound was his reforming influence on both general and forensic medicine in Britain (eg: R French and A Wear (eds), 1991, *British Medicine in an Age of Reform*. London & New York: Routledge).

4.6 William B. O'Shaughnessy, 1831, Poisoned Lozenges. *The Lancet* 2:192-198.

4.7 Ernest A. Gray, 1983, *By candlelight. The life of Dr Arthur Hill Hassall 1817-94.* London: Hale. This biography amplifies the necessarily brief summary in my text admirably.

4.8 Ernest A. Gray, 1983, as 4.7, p.87.

4.9 S.S. Sprigge, 1897, as 4.5.

4.10 O'Shaughnessy seems to have played little part in the Commission's subsequent work. Indeed, he cannot have had much spare time for it, despite being an impressively energetic Victorian. He spent most of his time in India, in the service of the East India Company as a Surgeon and as Assay Master of the Company's Calcutta Mint. These duties he combined with teaching at the Medical College of Calcutta, where he was Professor of Chemistry and Natural Philosophy, and also with overseeing the design and construction of the Indian Telegraph System on behalf of the Governor-General of Bengal. It was this latter business that brought him to England during 1851-53. In 1852 the Governor-General added Superintendent General of Telegraphs to his several posts. He had been elected a Fellow of the Royal Society of London in 1843 at the unusually young age of 34. Though trained in medicine, his professional interests included botany, medicinal chemistry, analysis and the newly emerging electrical science. In the 1830s he had designed an early form of telegraph himself, and his knighthood, conferred in 1856, was for services to electrical engineering. So distinguished a name was clearly an asset to Wakley's

Commission. [See A.F. Pollard, 1909, O'Shaughnessy, Sir William Brooke (1809-1889), *Dictionary of National Biography*, **14**:1305-5. London, Smith, Elder & Co; also J A Bridge, 1998, Sir William O'Shaughnessy, MD, FRS, FRCS, FSA: a biographical appreciation by an electrical engineer. *Notes Rec. R. Soc. Lond.* **52**(1):103-120.]

4.11 W.A.J. Archbold, 1909, Letheby, Henry (1816-1876) *Dictionary of National Biography*, 11:1010. London: Smith, Elder & Co.

4.12 A.H. Hassall, 1855, *Food and its Adulterations*. London: Longman, Brown, Green & Longmans. See also A H Hassall, 1857, *Adulteration Detected; or, Plain Instructions for the Discovery of Frauds in Food and Medicines*. Longman, Brown, Green, Longmans & Roberts. He consolidated both books in: A.H. Hassall, 1876, *Food, its Adulterations and the Methods for their Detection*. London: Longmans, Green & Co.

4.13 Anon., 1851, A chemical preventive force wanted. *Punch, or the London Charivari* 21:196.

4.14 Tom, Kingsley's boy hero, encounters evidence of "... foolish and wicked people who ... invent poisons for little children and sell them at wakes and tuck shops. Very well. Let them go on. Dr Letheby and Dr Hassall cannot catch them, though they are setting traps for them all day long." – Charles Kingsley, 1863, *The Water-Babies. A Fairy Tale for a Land-Baby*. (1890 edition, London: Macmillan, p.288).

4.15 Ernest A. Gray, 1983, as 4.7, p.108

4.16 W.F. Long, 1988, Dickens and the Adulteration of Food. *The Dickensian* (Autumn): 160-169.

4.17 J.A. Langford, 1887, as 0.4, vol. 1. pp. 9, 80ff, 97-98, 405.

4.18 Samuel Timmins, 1909, Scholefield, William (1809-1867). *Dictionary of National Biography*. 17: 910-911. London: Smith, Elder & Co.

4.19 J.A. Langford, 1887, as 0.4, vol.2, pp.446-447.

4.20 A contemporary issue of *The Lancet* reported that in March, 1854, the Birmingham Town Council had actually appointed a "public analyzer" to examine and suppress adulterations (Anon., 1854, Medical News. *The Lancet* (1) 293; see also E.W. Steib, 1966, as 0.2.). In all probability this report was mistaken. The Council lacked the power to make such an appointment until an enabling Act was passed several years later; it advertised the post soon after the Act in 1860.

4.21 J. Postgate and A.H. Browne, 1854, Adulteration of Food and Drugs. *The Lancet* (2) 492-493.

CHAPTER 5

5.1 Select Committee on Adulteration of Food, Drink and Drugs. 1885-6,

British Parliamentary Papers. Health: Food and Drugs Reports 1 and 2.
5.2 W.F. Long, 1988, as 4.16.
5.3 John Postgate, 1885-6, *British Parliamentary Papers. Health: Food and Drugs* **1**, Session 1885: Second Report from the Select Committee on Adulteration of Food, Drink and Drugs. Minutes of Evidence 2098-2134. (Postgate's oral evidence of 01/08/1855). Minutes of Evidence 2683-2754 (his oral evidence of 08/08/85). *ibid* **2**, Session 1886. Minutes of Evidence 4215-4386 (oral evidence and recommendations of 30/04/1856).

CHAPTER 6

6.1 J.A. Langford, 1887, as 0.4, vol.2, p.455.
6.2 Henry Morley, 1856, Poison. *Household Words* **XIII**:224-228 (22 March).
6.3 John Postgate, 1857, *A Few Words on Adulteration*. Birmingham: Billing's Steam-Press Offices.
6.4 B.T. Davis, 1967, as 0.6
6.5 John Postgate, 1857, as 6.3
6.6 John Postgate, 1857, On the Adulteration of Food and Drugs, and Mode of Prevention. *Trans. Nat. Assn. for the Promotion of Social Science*, p.483.
6.7 Anon., 1880, as 0.5
6.8 Anon., 1880, as 0.5
6.9 Report of letter, 1860, 'The Week', *Brit. Med. J.* 746.
6.10 J.A. Langford, 1857, as 0.4, vol.2, p.458.
6.11 J. Postgate, 1861, The Adulteration of Food and Drink Act. *Brit. Med. J.* 2: 241.
6.12 Anon., 1862, The Adulteration of Food *Brit. Med. J.* 1:123.
6.13 John Postgate, 1868, The Legislation on the Adulteration of Food, Drink and Drugs. *Trans. Nat. Assn. for the Promotion of Social Science* p.507.
6.14 J.A. Langford, 1857, as 0.4, vol.2, pp.463-464.
6.15 J.A. Langford, 1857, as 0.4, vol.2, pp.463-464.
6.16 J.A. Langford, 1857, as 0.4, vol.2, p.464.
6.17 Report from the Select Committee on Adulteration of Food Act (1872). Published 3 July 1874. *British Parliamentary Papers. Health: Food and Drugs* Reports 3.
6.18 Whitworth Jackson, 1874, as 6.17. Minutes of Evidence 3075-3076 (his oral evidence of 04/06/1874)
6.19 William Jackson, 1874, as 6.17. Minutes of Evidence 6673-6674. Also Robert Jackson, *ibid*, 6837-6839 (their oral evidence of 22/06/1874).
6.20 R.F. Giles, 1976, in: *Food Quality and Safety: A Century of Progress*. Symposium of the Ministry of Agriculture, Fisheries and Food. London: H M Stationery Office. pp.4-21.

CHAPTER 7

7.1 Scarborough Borough Council had no record in the mid 1980s of how it came by the portrait. It is likely, however, that it was donated by Postgate's son, Canon Langdale Horwood, in accordance with an instruction to that effect in his father's will. Langdale's estate also included a head-and-shoulders copy of Crome's portrait and a miniature of Postgate's wife Mary Ann; both have vanished.

7.2 Anon., 1880, as 0.5.

7.3 Was there a touch of irony in Postgate's allusion to debt? Trouble stemming from Sands Cox's administration had re-surfaced in 1859 and rumbled on until, in 1867, he was compelled to retire, leaving the college saddled with a debt of £10,000 (E.W. Vincent & D. Hinton, 1947, as 3.8).

7.4 John Postgate, 1862, An Introductory Address. in: W. Sands Cox, 1873, *Annals of Queen's College, Birmingham* **4**. pp.101-117. London: W.H. & L. Collingridge.

7.5 John Postgate, 1862, *Medical Services and Public Payments*. Untraced pamphlet, cited by Thomas Seccombe, 1909, as 2.7

7.6 John & Mary Postgate,1994, as 0.1, p.10.

7.7 Anon., 1880, as 0.5.

7.8 He moved from his original 80 Belmont Row (now an industrial yard), to 41 Frederick Street (an old wall of his garden is all that remained in 1998), probably around 1856; by 1868 his address was 59 Bristol Road (which still stands, probably much rebuilt), and at the time of his death he was living at Ferndale Villa, Pershore Road, in Edgbaston.

7.9 John Percival Postgate's wife, Edith, spoke thus of Isa Postgate to her youngest son Richmond, "Your Aunty Isa talks to the birds." She added cryptically, "But she's all right if she doesn't talk in a crowd." John Percival's elder daughter Margaret and his eldest son Raymond both regarded their Aunty Isa, in later life of course, as weak in the head. She was undoubtedly eccentric but, as so often in families of strong-minded individuals, prejudice again played some part: Margaret and Raymond were both rationalists, and Isa was intensely religious: she published at least seventeen booklets and poems among which nine extolled Christianity in a somewhat gushing style. Five other booklets, three of them poetry, did indeed deal with her friends the birds. Her booklets were mainly directed towards children, for whom she seems to have had a special feeling: in the early 1900s she sometimes looked after John Percival's three older offspring, while he and Edith had a holiday.

7.10 Isa Postgate, 1930, as 2.8.

7.11 There is a Flatfield House near Guiseley, Yorkshire, which could have inspired the name. Guiseley is remote from Driffield.

7.12 Margaret Cole, 1949, *Growing up into Revolution*. London: Longmans, Green & Co., p.4.
7.13 R.S. Conway, 1937, Postgate, John Percival. *Dictionary of National Biography* Oxford U. Press, pp. 685-6.
7.14 J.P. Postgate, 1909, *How to Pronounce Latin; a Few Words to Teachers and Others*. 3rd. ed. London: G Bell & Sons.
7.15 John & Mary Postgate, 1994, as 0.1
7.16 J.L. Postgate, 1881, *Umbrae: Poems and Translations*. Oxford: Thorntons.
7.17 Langdale Horwood Postgate was "impressively broad, rubicund and a little pompous" and could be seen "mounted on his formidable bicycle making stately progress through his parish" (See The Rev. R.P.W. Lanham, 1983-84, *The Ringing Grooves of Change*. Shillington: published privately in manuscript, pp. 45-47. Also Margery Roberts, 1986, Shillington, Past and Present (1), *Bedfordshire Magazine* XI, 253-261). His niece Margaret Cole (1949, as 7.8, p.4,fn) wrote of him:

> "... my uncle Langdale .... grew fat and amiable, and on the culmination of his black-covered paunch we used to watch, fascinated, a small gold cross swinging. He had a huge church very scantily filled, and his lady parishioners embroidered him slippers in purple."

Canon Langdale Postgate died in 1934, having been a widower for many years. In his will he bequeathed a sum of money to the humorous magazine *Punch* on condition that they supply free copies to a number of clergy in his diocese. The gift operated until the demise of Punch some 55 years later.
7.18 Anon., 1881, Obituary. *The Times*, September 30, p.9.
7.19 Anon., 1881, John Postgate, F.R.C.S., Birmingham. *Brit. Med. J.* 2:651.
7.20 Later the Warstone Lane Cemetery. There he had bought a plot for the burial of his daughter Mary Ann in 1857 and the grave was re-opened for his own interment. That area of the cemetery has since been flattened and no trace of their grave remains.

CHAPTER 8

8.1 Thomas Seccombe, 1909, as 2.7.
8.2 E.I. Carlyle, 1909, Thomas Wakley. *Dictionary of National Biography* **20**: 461-465. London: Smith, Elder & Co.
8.3 Anon., 1881, as 7.17.
8.4 Anon., 1881, as 7.18.
8.5 Anon., 1880, as 0.5.
8.6 T.D. Whittet, 1960, as 4.3.

8.7 Anon., 1881, untitled note. *The Lancet* 1:601.
8.8 Anon., 1881, Adulteration of Food and Drugs. *Lancet* 2:638-9.
8.9 S.S. Sprigge, 1897, as 4.5.
8.10 E.W. Steib, 1966, (as 0.2, p.307, fn.65) also commented on Hassall's unreliable view of his own accomplishments. In his autobiographical *Narrative of a Busy Life* (1893, London: Longman's & Co.) Hassall claimed to have been the first President of the Society of Public Analysts. In fact he was never President; that position was bestowed upon his stern critic Professor T. Redwood. Hassall was a Vice-President; apparently a notably inactive one.
8.11 Various authors, 1855, *The Lancet* **2**: 110-114.
8.12 Ernest A. Gray, 1983, as 4.7, p.108.
8.13 Ernest A. Gray, 1983, as 4.7, pp.106-7.
8.14 Anon., 1894, Arthur Hill Hassall, M.D.Lond. *The Lancet* **1**: 977-78.
8.15 T.D Whittet, 1960, as 4.3.
8.16 Ernest A. Gray, 1983, as 4.7, wrote, referring to Wakley and Hassall's exposures in *The Lancet*, "Ultimately the reports led to a meeting convened on 11 December 1854 by Mr J. Postage, F.R.C.S., of Birmingham..." (p.106).
8.17 G.K. Beeston, 1953, Brief History of the Inauguration of Food and Drug Legislation in Great Britain. *Food-Drug-Cosmetic Law J.* 8: 495-8.
8.18 E.W. Steib, 1966, as 0.2.
8.19 J. Burnett, 1989, as 4.4.

INDEX

(Illustrations have not been indexed, nor have entries in the Notes and References section)